Occupational Wholeness for Health and Well Being

T0225858

This practical book introduces a new, research-based *Model of Occupational Wholeness*, a way of conceptualizing *Satisfaction* with what one does to meet *one's Needs* for *Being, Belonging* and *Becoming*.

It explores how to conceptualize people's life stories through the model, take vital steps to help identify any problems, draw personal profiles, introduce intervention strategies for promoting *Well Being*. Focusing on enhancing *Well Being*, rather than ill health, the concept of *Occupational Wholeness* supports people to *Feel* more in *Control* of their own lives and helps to identify what *Balance* can be created, while recognizing *Personal* limitations and *Contextual* restrictions. Alongside theoretical background, it includes practice applications and practical tools, with scenarios and activities to consolidate learning. Providing a unique combination of the practice and theory of occupational science, Yazdani integrates occupational science, psychology and sociology with clinical experience of working with diverse groups of people in different countries.

This book is an important guide and reference for occupational therapists, occupational scientists, counsellors and life coaches.

Farzaneh Yazdani holds a BSc and MSc in Occupational Therapy from Iran University of Medical Sciences, Tehran. She started her professional life as a lecturer at Tehran's University of Social Welfare and Rehabilitation Sciences where she was also a clinician and practice educator in the field of Children and Mental Health Occupational Therapy. She established the first centre in the world for enhancing Well Being based on the model of human occupation in 1998 in Iran and received a commendation from the World Health Organisation (WHO). Her work in this centre led to Farzaneh receiving a visiting scholarship from the MOHO Clearing House, University of Illinois Chicago, by Professor Gary Kielhofner who supervised her PhD thesis along with Professor Musa Jibril, The University of Jordan. In 2000, Farzaneh was invited to help establish the Occupational Therapy department at The University of Jordan where she also achieved her MA in Psychological and Educational Counselling. Farzaneh joined Oxford Brookes University, UK in 2008 as a senior lecturer and currently works on her projects about sense of Being, Belonging and Becoming in two different population: 1- people diagnosed with Myalgia Encephalomyelitis (ME), 2- vulnerable immigrants, refugees and asylum seekers.

Niayesh Fekri is a multidisciplinary artist and educator. She graduated from the Slade School of Fine Art (UCL). Her art practice ranges from moving image, performance and writing. As an educator and facilitator, Niayesh works with art institutions to design and deliver workshops for young people and adults in community groups and educational settings.

Occupational Wholeness for Health and Well Being

A Guide to Re-thinking and Re-planning Life

Farzaneh Yazdani

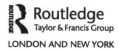
Routledge
Taylor & Francis Group

LONDON AND NEW YORK

First published 2023
by Routledge
4 Park Square, Milton Park, Abingdon, Oxon OX14 4RN

and by Routledge
605 Third Avenue, New York, NY 10158

Routledge is an imprint of the Taylor & Francis Group, an informa business

© 2023 Farzaneh Yazdani

British Library Cataloguing-in-Publication Data
A catalogue record for this book is available from the British Library

ISBN: 978-0-367-47299-3 (hbk)
ISBN: 978-0-367-47297-9 (pbk)
ISBN: 978-1-003-03475-9 (ebk)

DOI: 10.4324/9781003034759

Typeset in Bembo
by codeMantra

To my mother, Zari, who instilled love for humanity in me!

Contents

List of figures   ix
List of tables   xi
List of boxes   xiii
Foreword   xv
Preface   xix
Acknowledgements   xxi

1 Introduction: the underpinning knowledge of the Model of
   Occupational Wholeness   1
   FARZANEH YAZDANI AND NIAYESH FEKRI

2 The Model of Occupational Wholeness   14
   FARZANEH YAZDANI AND NIAYESH FEKRI

3 Understanding people and their narratives   34
   FARZANEH YAZDANI AND NIAYESH FEKRI

4 Identifying Incongruence/Gap, Disharmony   50
   FARZANEH YAZDANI AND NIAYESH FEKRI

5 Conceptualizing the Change that needs to be made   62
   FARZANEH YAZDANI AND NIAYESH FEKRI

6 Identifying the helpees' Readiness for Change (Change plan and
   implementation process)   71
   FARZANEH YAZDANI

7 Planning the Change   92
   FARZANEH YAZDANI

8 Implementing the strategies for Change   106
   FARZANEH YAZDANI

 9 Reflection as a strategy to enhance Self-Awareness   130
    FARZANEH YAZDANI

10 Applying the MOW in non–health-related settings   141
    FARZANEH YAZDANI AND NIAYESH FEKRI

11 Applying the MOW in in-patient and out-patient settings   159
    FARZANEH YAZDANI

12 The Occupational Wholeness Questionnaire   170
    FARZANEH YAZDANI

13 The MOW scholars and future directions of MOW projects   176
    FARZANEH YAZDANI

    Index   187

Figures

1.1	The MOW Hypothetical Triangle	11
2.1	The Hypothetical Triangle of Occupational Wholeness	15
2.2	The Hypothetical Actual and Ideal Triangles	27
4.1	Mary's Actual and Ideal Triangles	53
4.2	Ed's Actual and Ideal Triangles	54
4.3	Evan's Actual and Ideal Triangles	56
4.4	Zoya's Actual and Ideal Triangles	58
5.1	Simon's Scoring for his Actual and Ideal Triangles	67
5.2	Ayda's Actual and Ideal Triangles	68
6.1	Individual Intervention Decision–Making Chart	73
6.2	Scoring Triangle	76
6.3	Hanna's Triangles	84
6.4	Hanna's Intervention Decision–Making Chart	86
6.5	Public-level Decision-Making Chart	89
7.1	Change Process	93
7.2	Prediction/Expectation Card Board	99
8.1	Reversing Seats	108
8.2	Actual Being-Doings	108
8.3	Actual Belonging-Doings	109
8.4	Actual Becoming-Doings	109
8.5	Ideal Being-Doings	109
8.6	Ideal Belonging-Doings	110
8.7	Ideal Becoming-Doings	110
8.8	The Balloon Person	111
8.9	Feeling Cards	113
8.10	Thinking Cards	113
8.11	Doings Cards	114
8.12	Contextual Factors Cards	114
8.13	Expect–Predict Exploration Card Board	115
8.14	Devil–Angel Board	116
8.15	Change Motivators	117
8.16	The Feeling Wheel. Accessed at https://fosteractionohio.files.wordpress. com/2019/02/feeling-wheel.pdf–FIG_SRC	119
8.17	The Simplified Feeling Change Diagram	120
8.18	Example of a Like/Dislike Change form and Pie Chart	121
8.19	Doings Chart	122

8.20	Doing Chart Arita's Tailored Being-Doing Collage	123
8.21	Coping Box	124
8.22	What?, So What?, Now What? (3W) Diagram	125
8.23	Change Profile, Reflection on Feelings	126
8.24	Vignette Cards	127
8.25	Vignette Guide	128
10.1	The Wholeness Clock	149
10.2a	The Team Actual Triangle	153
10.2b	The Team Ideal Triangle	153
10.3a	Laura's First Art Piece at the Beginning of the Project	155
10.3b	Laura's Second Art Piece at the End of the Project	156
11.1	Althea's *Actual Triangle*, Disharmony and Incongruence	164
11.2	Analysis of the Need for Change for Althea	165
12.1	Changes in Rosa's OWQ II Scores	174
13.1	The MOW Network	177
13.2	The Occupational Wholeness Logo	177
13.3	Sarah Kufner	178
13.4	Mehdi Rezaee	180
13.5	Wa'd Abu Zurayk	181
13.6	Nadine Scholz-Schwärzler	182
13.7	Melissa Bowen	183
13.8	Laya Nobakht	184
13.9	Salma Nobakht	185
13.10	Niayesh Fekri	185

Tables

2.1	Contextual roles, definitions and examples	25
4.1	The MOW Concepts and Suggested Questions to Ask Helpees	51
6.1	The MOW Concepts in Lay Language	72
7.1	Being: Survival, Existing and Living Needs	95
7.2	Levels of Belonging	95
7.3	Aspects of Becoming Needs	96
7.4	Aspects of Change	98
7.5	A MOW-based Analysis of Sally's *Doings*	99
11.1	The MOW Concepts in Lay Language	161
12.1	Occupational Wholeness Questionnaire (OWQ) Version II	171
12.2	Rosa's OWQ II at Three Points: Prior to, Mid stage and after Two Weeks	173

Boxes

Box 1.1   Chapter aims   1
Box 1.2   Activities for learning and reflection   12
Box 2.1   Chapter aims   14
Box 2.2   Activities for learning and reflection   31
Box 3.1   Chapter aims   34
Box 3.2   Activities for learning and reflection   48
Box 4.1   Chapter aims   50
Box 4.2   Activities for learning and reflection   60
Box 5.1   Chapter aims   62
Box 5.2   Activities for learning and reflection   69
Box 6.1   Chapter aims   71
Box 6.2   Activities for learning and reflection   90
Box 7.1   Chapter aims   92
Box 7.2   Activities for learning and reflection   104
Box 8.1   Chapter aims   106
Box 8.2   Activities for learning and reflection   128
Box 9.1   Chapter aims   130
Box 9.2   Activities for learning and reflection   140
Box 10.1   Chapter aims   141
Box 10.2   Activities for learning and reflection   157
Box 11.1   Chapter aims   159
Box 11.2   Activities for learning and reflection   168
Box 12.1   Chapter aims   170
Box 13.1   Chapter aims   176
Box 13.2   Activities for learning and reflection   186

Foreword

After more than 100 years of establishing occupational therapy in the world, a limited number of theories in occupational therapy have developed for several reasons: First, development of the occupational therapy profession has required a history of research production and concept development. Looking back in occupational therapy history, it took over 70 years for the first well-structured model to be developed in occupational therapy by Gary Kielhofner in 1983. Since then, other models and theories have been developed in Western countries, which have shaped further the occupational therapy profession and led to its huge improvement. Second, developing theories requires talented, committed, multidimensional, experienced and exceptional people with a high-level, research-rich background that in a profession such as occupational therapy—which remains a scarce profession in nearly half the world's countries—is challenging. Third, developing a theory requires a supportive environment with access to related human and non-human resources. Even the Kawa model which is based on Japanese culture was developed by Michael Iwama who grew up, was educated, and worked in Canada and the USA (i.e., countries with several highly developed occupational therapy theories and models).

Culture is a prominent part of the occupational therapy theories and plays an important role in the process of evaluation and intervention. So, based on cultural and contextual differences, it is critical to have compatible models and theories that address people's needs within varied cultures. Almost all occupational therapy theories and models except the Kawa model originated from Western countries. Occupational therapy in Eastern countries is very young, with limited numbers of practitioners and related research. Therefore, occupational therapists in these countries have relied on Western occupational therapy theories and models to evaluate clients, develop management plans and implement interventions. As occupational therapy is culturally relevant, these Western models must be adapted to provide focused responses to the local needs, which is not ideal. Thus, the development of theories and models that better capture the needs, culture and preferences of Eastern people is critical.

Yazdani's work with the *Model of Occupational Wholeness* (MOW) is the first contribution by a person who grew up, trained and worked for most of her life in a Middle East country and the second within Asia. I met Dr Yazdani when she was my student in the final two years of her bachelor's degree in 1991, and I supervised her in a fieldwork placement in paediatrics. She was a very talented and exceptional student, with a high level of thinking and reasoning skills that were completely outstanding and different from other students whom I had taught so far. So, I knew that she would be very influential in the field of occupational therapy. Even I told her one time that she would be the first person to develop a model in Iran. Since then, we have become colleagues working in two countries and have continued our research with each other. I have witnessed how much she has immersed herself in the occupational therapy profession and how she has built and examined, piece by piece, this model over the past decades. I am sure that this model will open more doors for talented occupational therapy practitioners to build models in their countries based on their culture and context and enrich the occupational therapy profession across the globe.

Mehdi Rassafiani
Associate Professor, Charles Stuart University, Australia

In many ways, *MOW* offers an answer to a conundrum that has challenged me from the start of my training: How does the experience of what people do in their lives relate to the intervention approaches that are applied in occupational therapy? The development of occupational therapy as a clinical practice has tended to focus on individuals with medical conditions, who are often perceived as lacking a cultural context, a basis in a wider community, as well as an environment that determines so much of what they are able to do.

The *MOW* acknowledges these "unseen factors' contribution in shaping human actions" (Chapter 1, p. 9). *MOW* works with the unpredictability of change, the accidental and incidental events that were in my experience so important in working-class and community narratives. These events exposed people to circumstances but were also elements in their personal stories through which they achieved their understanding of the world and asserted their agency in it (Morley & Worpole, 2009; Woodin, 2018), directly or through their participation as a witness (Ragon, 1996), and perhaps as a survivor able to recognize how these events contributed to their sense of integrity (Ikiugu & Pollard, 2015). An outcome of these narratives of doing, being, becoming and belonging that many people may be able to relate to their family and peers—whether formally written as a testament or stories conveyed in a series of encounters—might be a sense of occupational wholeness.

This book presents a framework that can be applied across the diversity of communities and experiences—which as practitioners we may encounter—and thus may be particularly useful when working with people whose circumstances make them vulnerable. Through the use of the triangles in *MOW*, we can identify some of the discrepancies and disharmonies that may, through "helpers", be used as a basis to *Empower* people to form strategies leading to their own change, an approach towards their regaining *Control* of their circumstances. The breadth of its application may enable *MOW* concepts to complement the range of approaches developed by occupational therapists from the global south such as social occupational therapy (particularly with its emphasis on the quotidian experience; Lopes & Malfitano, 2020) and occupation-based community development (Galvaan & Peters, 2014). *MOW* also connects with southern occupational therapy's theoretical underpinnings that recognize personal engagement in transformation, such as Freire (1973), or else confront the invisibilities and marginalizations of epistemicide (de Sousa Santos, 2015). *MOW* therefore dovetails with other approaches developed by occupational therapists to work at a sustainable grass-roots level with individuals and communities.

Nicholas Pollard
Senior Lecturer, Sheffield Hallam University, UK.

The *MOW* details an occupational approach for working with people whose *actual* life does not match their perceived *ideal* life, leading to decreased satisfaction and wellbeing. Occupations, or human *Doing/Not Doing*, are positioned as the way for individuals to uncover a *tailored* (realistic) life that is closer to meeting their needs of being, belonging and becoming, thus improving their perception of wholeness. Although the *MOW* has its foundations in understandings of balance/imbalance, it shifts beyond perceiving these concepts as an objective dichotomy with the desired outcome of *balance*. Instead, it argues that *Doing/Not Doing* may need to be undertaken to meet one type of need that may contravene one's *Capacity* to meet another. The *MOW* approach focuses on understanding the subjective compromises and decisions that people must make to navigate the everyday "real" contexts of their occupational lives, which may necessitate periods of imbalance in occupational engagement to meet future wants, needs and expectations.

Although not explicitly stated, the *MOW* aligns with the philosophical approach of critical realism, which brings together ideas of agency and structure through its critiques of positivism and constructivism (Danermark et al., 2002). Critical realism highlights how unobservable social realities interact to expand or constrain, that is, privilege or oppress, certain people's access to occupations by shaping the occupational *Choices* and decisions people can or must make due to what is available to them. Although the *MOW*'s conceptualization of occupational engagement is different than my own, which does not require observable performance as part of its understanding (Davis, 2017), the *MOW* adds important considerations to working with people, who in their day-to-day lives must navigate multiple social identities based on the intersectionality of their social characteristics as experienced within overlapping systems that discriminate or disadvantage (Crenshaw, 1991).

The focus of the *MOW* on *Doing* and *Not Doing* offers a way of supporting changes in occupational engagement through a non-judgemental process by perceiving occupation as potentially both health-promoting and illness-producing regardless of the occupation. The *Choices* of *Doing/Not Doing* that people make can shape their lives in both positive and negative ways, thus having consequences for their wellbeing and wholeness. The *MOW* approach helps to increase awareness of one's realities, such as socio-cultural *Demands*, *Obligations*, systems of discrimination, as well as advantages, and the link between doing and satisfaction. Attributing value to *Doings* helps to identify and navigate the things that we must do that may not hold personal significance, but instead significance as a social or cultural *Expectations* or requirement, which acknowledges the real contexts in which our lives unfold. Thus, the *MOW* focuses on the intersecting domains of the real (social realities) and the actual and ideal *Doing/Not Doing* of individuals to support them in making compromises and decisions to support their wellbeing.

Jane A. Davis
Assistant Professor, University of Toronto, Canada

References

Crenshaw, K. (1991). Mapping the margins: Intersectionality, identity politics, and violence against women of color. *Stanford Law Review*, *43*(6), 1241–1299.

Danermark, B., Ekström, M., Jakobsen, L., & Karlsson, J. C. (2002). *Explaining society: An introduction to critical realism in the social sciences*. London: Routledge.

Davis, J. A. (2017). The Canadian Model of occupational performance and engagement (CMOP-E). In M. Curtin, M. E. Egan, & J. Adams (Eds.), *Occupational therapy for people experiencing illness, injury or impairment: Promoting occupation and participation* (7th ed., pp. 148–168). London: Elsevier.

Freire, P. (1973). *Pedagogy of the oppressed*. Harmondsworth: Penguin.

Galvaan, R., & Peters, L. (2014). *Occupation-based community development framework*. University of Cape Town. https://vula.uct.ac.za/access/content/group/9c29ba04–b1ee–49b9–8c85–9a468b556ce2/OBCDF/index.html, accessed May 2022.

Ikiugu, M., & Pollard, N. (2015). *Meaningful living through occupation*. London: Whiting and Birch.

Kielhofner, G. (1983). *Health through occupation. Theory and practice in occupational therapy*. Philadelphia, PA: F.A. Davis.

Lopes, R. E., & Malfitano, A. P. S. (Eds.) (2020). *Social occupational therapy: Theoretical and practical designs*. Edinburgh: Elsevier Health Sciences.

Morley, D., & Worpole, K. (Eds.) (2009). *Republic of letters* (2nd ed.). Philadelphia, PA/Syracuse: New City Communities Press/Syracuse University Press.

Ragon, M. (1996). *Histoire de la littérature proletarienne de langue français*. Paris: Albin Michel.

de Sousa Santos, B. (2015). *Epistemologies of the South: Justice against epistemicide*. Abingdon: Routledge.

Woodin, T. (2018). *Working-class writing and publishing in the late twentieth century: Literature, culture and community*. Manchester: Manchester University Press.

Preface

I was born into a family in which both my father and mother *Valued* hard work. That said, I was a teenager during the war between Iran and Iraq (1980–1989), when spiritual *Values* were talked about fervently and continuously at school, in the community and at home. While young men were defending the country at war zones, girls were *Expected* to study in order to *Become* skilful and educated to build the future of the country. Like many girls of my generation I was deeply influenced by these *Values*. For some, like me, with an ongoing health condition, I had to *Choose* where to spend my little energy. My decision was always education and work over other activities.

After completing my BSc and MSc in Occupational Therapy, I *Became* a young professional and my *Values* continued to dominate my time management with priority given to serious activities most of the time, over and above leisure and socializing. I was about 30 years old when invited to help with the establishment of an occupational therapy programme in Amman at the University of Jordan where I then stayed for more than eight years, studying for my second master's degree and Ph.D. in Psychological and Educational Psychology alongside working full time as a lecturer. It was only when invited to the Faculty of Rehabilitation, McGill University, Montreal, to speak on establishing the occupational therapy programme in Jordan, that I faced a *Reality* which made me *Think*.

While I was so proud of the hard work I had *Done* in Jordan, I suddenly *Felt* aware of the strange looks given by some of the audience, followed by some difficult questions. Why have you really gone so far without taking care of yourself? How about other aspects of your life? These questions became more entrenched in my mind when I moved to the UK and some of my colleagues used the term *Occupational Imbalance* to explain my lifestyle! I was so disappointed, as what I had *Thought* was the *Selflessness* of a young professional and academic who had contributed to *Do* big things such as helping establish several rehabilitation centres and programmes was considered by some people as madness and *Occupational Imbalance*.

I genuinely became interested in exploring what *Occupational Balance* really is and in my research I learned about life *Balance* as well. My initial thoughts of conducting a primary research project, therefore, cohered around exploration of the experiences and perspectives of occupational therapy practitioners and academics who use the term *Occupational Balance* in their field of work. A series of studies, of which some are published, led me to coin the term *Occupational Wholeness*. Becoming more familiar with the concepts underpinning occupational science, along with the findings of my studies, I realized that there is a gap between theoretical concepts and their application in practice in relation to Occupational Balance, Life Balance and *Occupational Wholeness*. Thus,

I proposed the *Model of Occupational Wholeness* that I have introduced in this book to help fill this gap.

While I have been an academic for 29 years, with experience of teaching in Iran, Jordan and the UK and led international workshops in different European and Middle Eastern countries, for the first 16 years I was also a practitioner. My other formal education and training, in the areas of educational and psychological counselling, also contributed to the content and structure of this book. Informed by the various strands of my background and thinking, I came to believe that the way a professional needs to think and formulate their ideas towards understanding a person who comes to them for help means that they are a professional helper and the person who looks for help is a helpee. These terms, helper and helpee, are used throughout this book.

While writing about my knowledge and experience provided a wonderful opportunity for *Reflection* on my professional and personal life, it was challenging to write in a second language and for a wide-ranging audience. As an Iranian academic who studied textbooks written in English and written mostly by scholars in Modern countries, I was very *Self-Aware* of how the *Contexts* of most textbooks were different from my own. I remember the difficulties I had in interpreting these books and applying them to my own teaching and education contexts. Throughout much of my academic life, I have had to educate my students about theories, concepts and models, along with their application, that had been formed in places which bore little similarity to my teaching context. I had to prepare my students to practise using knowledge that often differed from that which underlaid their usual practice. Concepts like *Self, Balance* and *Well Being* that have a different *Meaning* and *Value* in different *Contexts* and for different people were difficult for me to teach and for my students to understand. In writing this book, I thought of my readers, like my students, as being part of diverse social and political *Contexts* and I hope that this book encourages them and you alike to take the ideas presented here and translate them into your own personal and professional lifeworld and practice.

My daughter Niayesh who helped me to write several chapters raised my *Awareness* of many aspects of current global issues in relation to marginalized people. As a young artist with a vision about a diverse society and the rights of people from non-privileged backgrounds, she critically reviewed my chapters and scenarios and challenged my *Thinking* about diversity in my audience and beyond. I hope that feedback from my readers will help me to gain a deeper understanding of healthcare professionals working in other countries so as to enhance the quality of the *Model of Occupational Wholeness* and its utility in different *Contexts*.

Acknowledgements

I would like to thank the many people who supported me in their different capacities in the writing of this book.

Much is owed to my late father, *Ali*. Thank you for instilling in me a generous vision of the world.

I would like to thank all the helpees who agreed for their stories, directly or indirectly, to be shared and the scholars who contributed to the development of the *Model of Occupational Wholeness* by applying it and posing challenging questions.

I express my love and special thanks to my husband, *Dave*, whose experience in writing academic books inspired me. His support with my research and writing has been invaluable.

My siblings, *Afsaneh, Siamak, Soheila, Nastaran* and *Soheil*, have provided me with love, care and the spiritual energy I needed in hard times.

I also thank my friends, *Shiva* and *Chris*, for their care when I needed it.

And finally, my daughter, *Niayesh*. I wouldn't have been able to complete this book without you.

1 Introduction

The underpinning knowledge of the Model of Occupational Wholeness

Farzaneh Yazdani and Niayesh Fekri

Box 1.1 Chapter aims

This chapter will cover:

- *Balance* and *Imbalance* in an individual's life and their relationship with *Life Satisfaction* and *Self-Fulfilment*
- *Contextual Factors* contributing to individuals' *Choice-Making* and *Meaning-Making*
- The *MOW* views on *Life Balance and Satisfaction*, human *Needs, Choice* and *Meaning-Making* and the role of *Contextual Factors* on *Health* and *Well Being, Quality of Life*, and Significance of *Self-Awareness*
- The *MOW* aims

Human beings have always lived with several fundamental questions about themselves and their lives such as Who am I?, How should I live my life?, How much *Control* do I have over my life?, What can I do?, Where do I belong? and Who should I live or work with? Such questions appear throughout people's life. Although for much of the time, people become habituated to their life patterns and such questions may fade away until they are faced with a new situation that makes them *Reflect* on their position in regard to such questions. These new situations can be related to entering new life stages such as schooling, marriage and beginning a new job. They can also be related to unforeseen events such as illness, accidents, bankruptcy and the like. For some people, such questions are not important or pressing. People whose lives are dictated by the struggle to obtain basic survival *Needs*, for example, may not have the time to mindfully address or even entertain such questions. Others may have the time, yet they may not have the language to frame or express them. However, even in the most minute and simplest forms, these questions still exist.

In the process of human development, people encounter new things to deal with, more ways to deal with them and from this ongoing process, new questions arise as to how to manage them all. This process can be seen in the early stages of life when a child develops the ability to move around independently. As the child takes new steps, they discover their own *Capacities* and more of the world around them: how to comprehend it and how to interact with it. In everyday situations, people try to keep a *Balance* amongst the varying aspects of their lives. For instance, *Choosing* to watch TV and being

DOI: 10.4324/9781003034759-1

required to do homework are two uses of a child's time which meet their *Need* for enjoyment and their *Need* for learning and progressing their future. A child may require to *Balance* these two *Needs* in their life, and caregivers usually support children in learning how to *Balance* these aspects of their lives. *Balance* and *Imbalance* can be viewed at a variety of time scales: daily, weekly, yearly and so on.

The *Model of Occupational Wholeness* (*MOW*) introduced in this book has developed from a body of research into the concept of *Occupational Balance* which has led to the emergence of a new concept called *Occupational Wholeness* (*OW*). *Occupational Wholeness* looks into human *Occupational Balance* from a different perspective. In order to understand the background of the *MOW*, this chapter provides an outline/history of/a discussion of the existing knowledge related to the fundamental concepts underpinning the *MOW*.

Life Balance

The issue of *Balance* in human life can be looked into from several perspectives. At the most basic level, human biology seeks *Balance* in its processes and functions. From the smallest of cells to the body's biological clock, the mechanisms within these components of human biology are embodiments of *Balancing* processes at the behavioural level. People may refer to *Balance* when there is no tension between the tasks, roles and *Responsibilities* they have in their life. According to Carlson et al. (2009) and Kofodimos (1993), *Balance* requires a '*Balancing* act'—an ongoing exercise of juggling multiple demands and *Responsibilities*. People continually move between *Balance* and *Imbalance*, and as a consequence they need to manage the ongoing *Changes* between the two. *Imbalance* is a natural occurrence in the process of seeking to *Satisfy Needs*, *Wants* or desires. Many people do not have the opportunity to live their lives according to their desires and *Wants* when they are caught up with securing basic survival *Needs*. In other words, survival *Needs*, such as exchanging labour for resources, come before the *Wants* when making *Choices* about what to *Do*. *Needs* are indispensable, although some are more obvious than others such as the *Need* for sustenance. There is a further layer of basic *Needs* such as the human *Need* for *Autonomy*. *Wants* on the other hand are what a person desires but can live without. While *Wants* may contribute to the quality of life, at times a pseudo *Need* may be created that must be met; otherwise, the consequent disappointment can result in psychological issues. The pseudo *Needs* are consequences of the modern world that spreads the idea of *Happiness* tied up with a particular lifestyle. For instance, some companies flow a variety of products that suit these kinds of lifestyles that create a pseudo *Need* that is a *Need* that is created artificially. Some people, then, *Think* they should get them to ensure their *Happiness*. The expansion of desires, preferences and, at times, opportunities has led to further development of what is perceived as *Need* based on what people seek for a better quality of life. As such, rapid and continuous *Changes* in society have affected the extent and complexity of human *Needs* and *Wants*, creating *Gaps* between what people *Need*, their *Capacities* and the opportunities that are available to them. Consequently, discrepancies between people's *Needs* and *Wants* present a continual conflict that can lead to *Dissatisfaction* regardless of the extent of people's material or economic resources (Alderfer, 1969; Fitzgerald, 2016).

Approaches to *Balance* and *Imbalance* vary in the factors they designate as needing to be *Balanced*, for instance *Balancing* family and work, different roles that people play,

Needs and *Wants* and daily activities (Matuska et al., 2013). Within these approaches are occupational scientists' specific view of *Balance* and *Imbalance* in what people *Do* which is known as occupation. The authors' initial research on the concept of *Occupational Balance* led to the development of concept of *Occupational Wholeness* that introduces a form of *Balance* explained as *Harmony* amongst the three *Needs*: *Being*, *Belonging* and *Becoming* expressed through *Doings* which are explained in detail in this book (Yazdani & Bonsaksen, 2017; Yazdani et al., 2016).

Life Satisfaction and Happiness

Satisfaction with Life has been theorized and studied for decades, and there is a variety of views on what contributes to people's evaluation of their life and subsequent *Feelings* of *Satisfaction* or *Dissatisfaction* with it. These theories have either looked at the issue of *Life Satisfaction* as an evaluation of an individual's overall life in general or from a certain viewpoint within a specific domain. Examples of the latter are investigations into *Satisfaction* regarding work, finance, family or *Health* (Cummins, 2005). The most researched theories in explaining the sense of *Satisfaction with Life* seem to be the ones that have looked at the issue through a domain-specific lens. Studies based on these theories have found that some categories/types of domain-specific *Satisfaction* lead to an overall sense of *Satisfaction* with life, although there is a difference in the level that each domain contributes to global *Life Satisfaction* (Loewe et al., 2014).

According to the Whole *Life Satisfaction* theory of *Happiness*, people are *Happy* when they make the judgement that their life fulfils their ideal life-plan (Feldman, 2008). The emphasis on the ideal situation has raised critique as it seems to be *Unrealistic* or un-achievable for most people. Suikkanen's (2011) approach to *Life Satisfaction* supports the idea that individuals *Need* to be helped in the way they formulate their ideals. Therefore, people can be *Happy* with a more *Realistic* view of themselves when comparing their *Actual* and hypothetical *Self*, life or situation.

It is also important to consider the difference between the two terms: *Satisfaction* and *Happiness*. *Life Satisfaction* is a cognitive process of an individual's evaluation of themself and/or their life, while *Happiness* refers to a *Feeling* which may come and go in a period of time. *Happiness* is a subjective experience that may or may not be associated with *Life Satisfaction* (Diener et al., 1999). These perspectives mean that individuals may evaluate their own situation as *Satisfactory* yet *Feel Unhappy* as their subjective experience is not positive. Put in another way, *Happiness* is a *Feeling*, and some people seldom experience it even in the presence of a positive cognitive evaluation of their life situation.

Life Balance and Satisfaction from the perspective of the MOW

The author's perspective on the matter of *Life Balance/Imbalance* and *Life Satisfaction* as an occupational therapist links to the significance of people's *Doings* in order to meet their *Being*, *Belonging and Becoming Needs* in their own *Context*. *Balancing* and *Imbalancing* are processes in which an individual survives, exists and evolves. *Balance* and/or *Imbalance* are relative concepts that rely on individuals' perspective of themselves and their situation. Regardless of people' *Individual Capacities* and *Contextual* resources, many have little time to spend on *Thinking* through what they are *Doing* or *Not Doing* which affects *Balance* and/or *Imbalance* in their lives. In other words, those fundamental questions mentioned at the beginning of the chapter may not be at the forefront of a person's *Awareness* at different periods of their life. Consequently, how they *Think* and *Feel* about what they *Do* and what they *Need* becomes habitual and less reviewed. The ways of living and surviving under the demands of modern life do not necessarily allow time for *Re-thinking* and *Reflecting* on individuals' actions within their life situations. People who are socio-economically disadvantaged or live under politically unstable circumstances must create survival strategies. On the other hand, the very rich and elite use their power to exploit those less fortunate than themselves so that only the pseudo *Needs* which they have created for themselves can be fulfilled. A variety of resources is needed to attain the ever-inflating standard of welfare and luxury set by those with socio-economic privilege. Here, a *Gap* begins to form between an *Individual's Capacity*, their *Contexts* or opportunities and the dreams and aspirations they have.

The *MOW* proposes that although *Balancing* individuals' *Doings* aids a sense of fulfilment with *Self* and their life, it may not necessarily ensure good mental/physical Health. *Subjective Well Being (SWB)* and *Life Satisfaction* are more related to *Balancing* and at times *Imbalancing Doings*. This means that *Imbalancing* is necessary for meeting people's *Needs* of *Being*, *Belonging* and *Becoming*. These concepts are explained in Chapter 2, where the *MOW* is presented in detail. According to the *MOW*, at times, lack of *Balance* is a natural part of a person's life that aids their *Satisfaction with Life* and themself. In some situations, *Imbalance* is necessary for a period of time in order to achieve *Balance* at another period of time. While some people may actively force *Imbalance* in their lives, others may only encounter *Imbalance* due to the transition between different stages of their life. Passive or active, people perpetually face *Balance* and *Imbalance* through their lifetime. Therefore, *Imbalance* may be a natural event in life or people may *Choose* it intentionally to meet some aspects of their *Needs* and consequently *Feel Satisfaction*. Therefore, *Imbalance* in life does not always have negative implications for people's *Health* or *Well Being*. It can even support an individual's sense of *OW* which is explained in more depth in the next chapter.

The MOW and human Needs

Occupational scientists believe that the human is an occupational being who meets their *Needs* through *Doing* (Wilcock, 2007). There are different views as to what human *Needs* are, what shapes them and how they shape actions. People *Do* a variety of things in their day-to-day life (what is called occupation in occupational science terminology) to meet their *Needs*. People also intend *Not to Do* at times and *Not Doing* should be equally looked into when studying human occupation. For this reason, the word *Doings* is used in this book to include both *Doing* and *Not Doing*. At times, individuals try to create *Harmony* between what they *Do/Not Do* in order to meet their *Needs*. However, this is not always successful. The *MOW* divides human *Needs* into three fundamental *Needs* related to the senses of *Being, Belonging* and *Becoming* that are met through people's *Doings*. From this perspective, occupational scientists discuss the variety of occupations and different things that individuals *DO* to ensure *Balance* for *Health* and/or *Well Being* (Wilcock, 2007).

Choice-Making and Meaning-Making and the role of Context

People indicate if their life is in *Balance* or *Imbalance* and then *Attribute Value* to that *Balance* or *Imbalance*. For instance, an individual may say that *Changing* jobs *Imbalanced* their life, but that they are *Happy* about it as this *Imbalance* has forced them to educate themself and learn new skills which will help their future. To this person, *Imbalance* means opportunity and is *Attributed* as a positive *Value*. Another person may see job *Changing* as an unfortunate situation that has caused them lots of effort in learning new skills, taking up their time. For this person, *Changing* jobs means stress which may be considered as a negative *Value*. The *Meaning* and *Value* people give to events depend on their individual characteristics and the *Context* they live in. At times, people may give positive *Meaning* or *Value* to things that have no bearing on their *Health, Well Being*, growth, *Life Satisfaction* and *Happiness*. For instance, to a teenager, drug use may be viewed as an act of exercising *Autonomy* even if it has harmful effects on their *Health* and other aspects of their life. Yet, it's also important to note that not all teenagers perceive drug use in such a way. A positive *Meaning Assignment* to drug use is based on the teenager's individual characteristics as well as their social and economic environment, friends in particular. There are always several personal and *Contextual Factors* that contribute to *Meaning-Making*. The *Context* of a person's life influences their beliefs about the causes of their actions and their outcomes. *Contextual Factors* influence a person's view of themself and their world and the way these two interact. *Contextual Factors* consist of the real and virtual environments that people live in. The intersection of geographical, temporal, institutional, political, socio-economic and physical factors is the main influence in the process of *Meaning-Making* that interacts with people's individual characteristics and *Capacities*. Social influences have become even more complicated since the Internet has made social media sites and advertising increasingly more accessible. An increasingly diverse range of social influences are infiltrating people's everyday lives, as such the parameters of the influence of people's social surroundings are also broadened both in terms of time and space. In other words, there are many individuals who are exposed to a vast range of options without *Realistically* having access to them. The virtual world's influence on people's life has become extremely prominent. Through the virtual world, making *Choices* and practising *Autonomy* are encouraged, the truth of what 'options' and '*Choices*' are *Really* available is confused. For instance, take environmental activism, an important issue which has been co-opted by social media trends. Many environmentally conscious online celebrities in Europe and the US advocate actions which are specific to the structures within which they live. As such, for many in the world, the environmental activism advocated online is dominated by ideals which are difficult at best, or impossible to achieve. For example, for people who live in a country that doesn't have an infrastructure for recycling, or cannot access ethically sourced goods, these social ideals of ethical living become a luxury that can be attained by the very few and subsequently they become a sign of wealth. Thus, an inflation in the variety of social influences through social media has meant that individuals are exposed to increasingly unrealistic options. In practice, however, many of these social influences are unattainable to many who seek them. The intersection of the individual's economic, social and political *Context* and their ethnicity, gender and sexuality and so on make it difficult, if not impossible, to identify a cause-and-effect relationship between individual factors. It is true that social media has also allowed individuals to be part of social/community groups which are not restricted geographically. This has meant that they can form connections with others across the world based on their interests and/or beliefs. On the other hand, confusion may arise from being part of several social/community groups which may have different priorities or even contradicting ones. This phenomenon of overexposure perceived as *Choice* can lead to problems in people's beliefs about their own capabilities, to misjudgements about their resources and to *Dissatisfaction* or *Unhappiness*. Another aspect of this overexposure presents itself in how individuals *Feel* in relation to matters that are out of their *Control*. An example of this can be seen in the issues that arose during the 2020 Covid-19 pandemic. As various governments and *Health* departments took different approaches to enforcing isolation measures, many individuals became acutely *Aware* of their helplessness in such a situation. Exposure to all the different beliefs and information about how to handle the spread of this virus may have had an effect on the *Choices* people made to keep safe; however, ultimately the protocols enforced by the authorities were the ones by which people had to abide.

Assigning Meaning, making *Choices* and *Attributing Values* to these decisions about X and Y affect an individual's sense of *Control* over themselves and their world and consequently their *Satisfaction* of self. Hence, people's *Self-Fulfilment* is dependent not only on what they *Do or Not Do* but also on the way they process *Meaning, Choice* and *Values* regarding their *Doings*.

Bringing together all the above factors that link peoples' *Doings*, namely *Balance* and *Imbalance*, sense of *Self-Fulfilment* and overall *Satisfaction* with *Life* and *Choice* and *Meaning-Making* are the basic blocks of the concept of the *MOW*. The *MOW* tries to facilitate developing and enhancing the individual's *Awareness* about their *Doings* and their association with their *Actual* and *Ideal* life situation. The *MOW* tries to aid people in making the best of their opportunities and managing their limitations so as to help shape a sense of personal *Fulfilment* and *Satisfaction* with their *Life*.

According to the *MOW*, people are required to make *Changes* to their *Actual* situation and the way they *Think* about their *Ideal* if they are looking for *Satisfaction with Life* and a sense of *Self-Fulfilment*. The first step in making *Change* is identifying what requires *Changing* and being *Motivated* to take action towards *Change*. A variety of factors take part in the *Motivation* for action. People may *Feel Motivated* to take action if they *Think* what and how they *Do* or *Not Do* can *Change* their situation. The level of *Control* people believe they have over a situation is significant in *Motivating* or *Demotivating* them into taking action for making *Change*. People may ascribe the cause of their actions and life events to external or internal factors, and this is associated with the level of *Control* they assume they have on the occurrence of events and their own actions (Weiner, 1972). People's views on the causality of events or their own actions and the level of *Control* they may *Feel* over a situation can help in *Predicting* whether they take any action to *Change* their life situation or not. External ascribing of causes for events, when people believe they have little or no *Control* over them, doesn't *Motivate* the person to take any action towards making *Change*. Internal ascription for causes of actions and events, on the other hand, refers to factors from within an individual. Other characteristics of the influential factors or causes of an event that affect people's *Motivation* for action towards changing them are related to the *Changeability* of those factors and how the individual perceives the possibility of *Change* in those factors. For instance, if an individual believes in luck as a factor that can determine success in an exam and considers that luck is not *Changeable* but predetermined, the individual would not be *Motivated* towards influencing the outcome of their exam. Whether these factors cause or influence an event is affected by the way people *Feel* they have *Control* to influence or *Change* them. The perspective on influencing factors in *Controlling* an act or event leads to a very different *Motivation* for action and perceptions of the individual engaging in a process of making

Change (Rotter, 1990). Later in this book, the authors discuss how the intervention that helpers put in place with and for helpees depends on the way helpees perceive their ability to influence *Change* in their life. This ascription of causality and sense of *Control* on action and life situation plays a significant role in initiating action. Rotter (1966) introduced the concept of the locus of *Control* that refers to an individual's perception about the main underlying causes of events. Later, Zimbardo (1985) explained that the orientation of belief about the outcomes of people's action relies on internal *Control* from within a person or on events outside personal *Control*. A biased ascription of causality to either *Self* or environment may lead to *Unrealistic Expectations*. An exaggerated locus of *Control* in either direction may affect people's *Well Being*. People may consider a strong internal locus of *Control* and personalize responsibility for actions or events over which they have no *Control* or *Choose* that they must pay a high price in order to take *Control* over their action. People with an exaggerated internal locus of *Control* may personalize *Responsibilities* for every event without considering others' *Responsibilities* in those events, and this can harm their self-esteem, leading to self-guilt, self-blame and even depression. Equally, not taking any responsibility for events when they should is seen in people with an extreme external locus of *Control* that can lead to blaming others and *Feeling* like a victim and potentially lead to depression too. It is important to ascertain how much *Control* people assume they have over their situations, and how much *Change* they may be able to instill. The ascription of causality, if *Unrealistic*, can lead to psychological distress, *Life Dissatisfaction* and *Unhappiness*. It is inevitable that people have limited knowledge and experience in understanding their own and others' behaviour and make assumptions that, in turn, may lead to undesired results. For instance, an individual may assume that success is achieved only through hard work and dismisses the impact of their capability and extraneous factors. For this person, putting a lot of effort in *Doing* things for which they may not have capability may not bring success and therefore lead to *Dissatisfaction* with themself and their *Life*. Understanding the cause and effect of people's actions and consequences is oversimplified when reduced to what is observed or perceived at the time of the event without acknowledging the impact of previous events on the matter. Another example of oversimplifying cause and effect in human behaviour is when an individual's action is overgeneralized within a cultural *Context*. For instance, in some cultures, gender-related characteristics are too generalized, and the cause of an individual's behaviour may be reduced to a gendered stereotype and overlooked.

The above discussion and examples illustrate the complexity of how individuals perceive their own action as their own *Choice*, as having *Control* over it and being able to *Change* it or not. Therefore, in a process of aiding *Change* in anyone's life, there is a need to understand how they perceive things, their potential biases and the extent to which they can *Change* their attitudes and beliefs. This understanding is crucial in a helper-helpee relationship to establish common ground for further action towards potential *Change*. Without in-depth understanding, the helping intervention may be unsuccessful. Learning what the sources of *Motivation* for an individual's action are and to what extent they *Feel Motivated* and able to invest in *Change* is essential in building an intervention.

The MOW, Health and WellBeing

One of the main changes that seemed necessary in recent decades was to aid people as individuals or communities to move towards better *Health*. In the last three decades, promoting *Health* has become one of the aims of governments in many countries (WHO, 2021). However, issues around mental illness and psychological distress, lower *Life Satisfaction* and poorer *Subjective Well Being* have only recently attracted the attention of scholars in the field health promotion (WHO, 2021). With rapid *Changes* in the world, in technology in particular, lifestyles seem to be the subject of dramatic *Change*. Such *Change* happens as demands in life keep snowballing, and it seems hard to keep up with everything. People are forced to adapt to the *Changes* in their way of life as formulated at a political level yet act on the basis of the demands placed on them by their surroundings.

People's belief about themselves and how they *Feel Satisfied* with their own "*Self*" and "world" are fundamental aspects that shape their *Subjective Well Being*. *Awareness* about the relationship between an individual's belief and *Value* system and how they interact is a key element of *Change*. The link between human *Emotion* and cognition, regardless of the causal relation between them, shows how understanding *Health* / ill *Health* is not enough for perceiving *Well Being*. People could be objectively *Healthy* and consider themselves *Healthy*, but not necessarily *Feel Healthy*. Overall sense of contentment is not achieved unless people first recognize their life situation and then address whether what they might *Do/Not Do* is literally what they had planned or hoped for. A sense of *Harmony* between a person and their world is the core of human *Satisfaction with Life and Self-Fulfilment*: *Feeling* as *Whole* and as one piece (Yazdani & Bonsaksen, 2017).

The MOW and (people's views on the) Quality of Life

Based on the *MOW,* people's views on their quality of life and what gives them a sense of *Self-Fulfilment* are essential to their *Subjective Well Being*. As mentioned earlier in this chapter, people's perception of what it means to live a good quality of life is influenced heavily by the *Context* in which they live. While some people may have clearer ideas about a good quality of life, others may be confused due to over- or under-exposure to life opportunities, options and perhaps *Choices* that they may or may not have.

Significance of Self-Awareness

Another important aspect of human *Satisfaction with Life* and a sense of *Self-Fulfilment* depends on the level of *Awareness* that individuals have about themselves and their *Context*. People may *Feel* and *Think* about their everyday life experiences or be inspired by things that are not necessarily known to them.

Confronting people with some *Realities* about their own *Thoughts* and *Feelings*, and *Doing* so at times when they are not *Happy* with themselves and their life, could be a very challenging situation for both helpers and helpees. However, Duval and Wicklund (1972) when introducing the idea of objective *Self-Awareness* highlighted its significance as the key to *Change*. People are more likely to align their behaviour with their standards when made *Self-Aware*. The authors argue that *Self-Awareness* is not just about *Changing* what people *Do* to move towards their *Values* and standards but also inviting them to *Reflect* on their *Values* and standards too as they may require *Change*. According to Bandura (2012), that people's belief about their capability to organize and execute the courses of action necessitates *Self-Awareness*. The *MOW* adds that *Awareness* about people's *Context* and its interaction with *Self* is essential for *Change* in *Doings*. Although to be able to make a clear distinction between what people can *Do* about their life and the way others have impacted on it requires understanding of *Self* before the *Context, Being*

Aware of what people *Do* with their time and energy *Empowers* them to *Make Choices* that could bring more *Satisfaction* to their lives. Contemporary life's fast-*Changing* nature makes it harder for such *Awareness* to occur.

Challenging Personal and Contextual circumstances and Self-Awareness

When the *Context* challenges what a person may consider as 'normal', everyday life becomes more complicated. For example, when a child is born with an impairment, several aspects of their *Doings* could face challenges. The formation of the child's *'Being'* is influenced by their familiarity with and experience of people around them in their life. When the *Context* (people or places) is unfamiliar to the child's situation (for instance, a child with visual impairment), the child may find it difficult to comprehend what they can or cannot do in a *Context* of all visually intact people. Parents' knowledge of parenting is generally based on their own childhood experiences and from other parents' experiences. Having a child with an impairment or disability may not be what they have seen and learned about before. Being unfamiliar can cause misunderstanding, as many people use their own experiences as an initial reference point for understanding others. Even when others try to understand what the child with an impairment can/cannot *Do*, they have fewer ideas about the child's *Being, Belonging* and *Becoming* (Ho, 2008; Robinson & Notara, 2015; Stephens et al., 2015). Neglecting the *Needs* of a child with an impairment plays a significant role in changing an impairment into a disabling situation. Basic psychological *Needs* such as *Autonomy*, competence and affiliation play an essential role in meeting *Being, Belonging* and *Becoming Needs* and require attention in ensuring a person's mental *Health* and psychological growth (Clayton et al., 2013). In many cases, basic conditions for survival often become the focus of others' attention when it comes to planning services for people with disabilities. Impairment at any stage of an individual's life has an impact on their perceived *'Being'*. Finding time to be mindful of how individuals are spending their own time and energy has proven to be difficult for many, in particular when their life situation gets hard. For people with *Health* issues, finding time is even more complex because of the mental and physical energy that goes into dealing with their *Health* issues and the impact of them on their lives. Any *Change* in life, including natural *Change* due to development and growth, means that human beings are in a constant state of *Imbalance* or *Balance*. For people who *Think* life is about reaching a static *Balance*, this ongoing *Change* could create distress by leaving them to *Feel* that something is always missing or out of place.

What the MOW aims to achieve

The *MOW* tries to aid helpees (the individual) to have a better understanding of their *self*, their *Context* and the interaction of the two in shaping people's sense of *Being, Belonging* and *Becoming* and *Doings*. Individuals develop a sense of fulfilment based on *Harmony* between their *Needs* and the way they meet them. Identifying every individual sense of *Harmony* relates to the right combination of *Doings* that can fulfil all aspects of an individual's existence that is about who they are and will be in connection with and relation to their *Context*. For example, for a person with limited cognitive, *Emotional* and physical *Capacity,* the right combination of *Doings* could be restricted to their personal and *Contextual Capacities*. What they can *Do* might be restricted due to limited

Capacities. However, they still could identify a right combination of *Doings* to meet their *Needs* for *Being, Belonging* and *Becoming* and not just on a survival level. This means even an individual with the most limited *Capacity* could still connect to time, space and people in a fair world to achieve their sense of *OW.*

The *MOW* intervention is based on making *Changes* in people's *Doings.* Skar (2004) states that human beings as organic dynamic systems are able to *Change* and adapt their environment as well as themselves. He argues that there is a high level of complexity in interaction between humans and their surroundings that makes the identification of cause and effect in human behaviour uncertain. Acknowledging the complexity of the cause-and-effect relationship, however, does not contradict the associative relationship between factors from within and outside individuals. The significant point of consideration is to validate the nonlinear relationship between human behaviour and the contributing factors, acknowledging the unseen factors' contribution in shaping human actions. This does not mean that there is no potential for *Predicting* the consequences of a person's actions that may appear to be very disappointing and frustrating, as well as *Devaluing* of, the person's *Control* over themself and their life. *Prediction* of the consequences of *Change* is another determining factor to *Motivation* for action towards *Change* besides what were discussed as contributing factors to *Motivation* for action earlier in this chapter. Life is a series of hypotheses that each individual puts in place and tests with some evidence that supports or hinders the outcomes in one way or another. History and science have supported some of these hypotheses more than the others, and this is the reason for a lot of similarities in human experiences and the so-called cause-and-effect relationships that appear to have strong *Predictor* values. Therefore, in spite of complex relationships amongst indefinite factors in the world, there is still potential for the *Prediction* of human action and its consequences, particularly at an individual level. The role of helpers therefore is to facilitate developing hypotheses and testing them for people who require help from others. Considering the characteristics of individuals and their *Contextual* contribution to people's sense of *Wholeness* as a dynamic system justifies a role for some people as helpers. Considering human beings as a dynamic system, making *Change* in any part of this system *Changes* other parts (Lehman et al., 2017). Within the context of the *MOW,* helpers can assist people to make *Changes* in and of the *MOW* components and *Expect Change* in other components, although this *Change* is not always *Predictable.* The complexity of humans in this complex world, however, requires evaluating cause and effect within their lives again and again. As chaos theory posits that events do not always unfold in a *Predictable* way (Duke, 1994). Therefore, *Reflecting* on an individual's action and its consequences is an essential part of interventions.

The rest of this book presents ideas about how helpers can help people to understand themselves and their own *Contexts* so as to assist them in making *Changes* in places and at times so that the helpee might reach their potential and achieve their own level of *OW.* As *Change* in people's *Context* also plays a significant role in their *Choices* and *Doings,* facilitating *Change* for individuals is an indispensable role of authorities and governments. Hence, a crucial part of helpers' duties is to advocate for the *Changes* required on an individual and public level.

The MOW and its Triangles

The *MOW* components and their relationships are presented as *Triangles.* These *Triangles* are used to aid helpers' and helpees' communication through visualizing the *MOW*

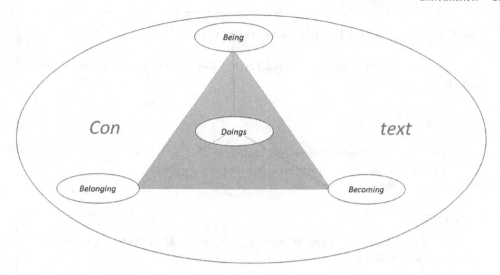

Figure 1.1 The MOW Hypothetical Triangle

concepts. In this chapter, only the hypothetical *Triangle* surrounded by *Contextual Factors* in a circle that illustrates the main *MOW* perspective is introduced (see Figure 1.1).

Doings is the central point of the triangle and the *Context* that demonstrates the links between *Being, Belonging* and *Becoming*. Chapter 2 expands on the concepts of *Doings* and sense of *Being, Belonging* and *Becoming* in relation to *Context* and how they are linked as a *Triangle* within a circle. This *Triangle* is referred to as the *3Bs* of *Doings*.

Summary

Inquiry into *Occupational* and *Life Balance* initiated a series of studies that led to the concept of *OW*. The authors employed several theories and approaches to explain her findings. Of those, the dynamic system theory, chaos theory, needs theories, attribution theories, theories of behaviour change, *Self* theories and theories of occupational science were the most significant that guided the authors' thoughts: analysis and synthesis of the *MOW*. The author's journey started from a question about what *Occupational* and *Life Balance* mean to people and healthcare professionals, in particular occupational therapists. The term *Wholeness* then seemed to be more efficient in explaining what people mean by *Balance*. The fundamental components of the *MOW* were identified as the *3Bs*: *Being, Belonging* and *Becoming* as human *Needs* that are met through *Doing/Not Doing* in the human *Context*. *Context* therefore necessitates further exploration for its interaction with and impact on the *3Bs* and human *Doings* that consist of what an individual might intentionally and voluntarily *Do* or *Not Do*. To explain the contributing factors in *Doings* and their link to other components, the role of *Choice-Making* and *Meaning-Making* for an individual's own actions and life events were explained. The ascription of causality also explained human *Motivation* for action. *Life Satisfaction* and *Self-Fulfilment* were discussed in relation to the sense of *OW* and its association with *Subjective Well Being*. This basic knowledge is presented in brief to set the background for Chapter 2 about the components of the *MOW* in detail.

Box 1.2 Activities for learning and reflection

These activities are set to help you think further about the topics presented in this chapter.

Activity 1:

- What makes you *Feel Satisfied* with your life?
- What do you *Do* to give yourself a sense of *Self-Fulfilment*?

Activity 2:

- In your own language, explain what the aim of the *MOW* is to someone who doesn't know about the *MOW*.

References

Alderfer, C. (1969, May). An empirical test of a new theory of human needs. *Organizational Behavior and Human Performance, 4*(2), 142–175.

Bandura, A. (2012). *On the functional properties of perceived self-efficacy revisited* (vol. 38, pp. 9–44). Los Angeles, CA: Sage Publications:.

Carlson, D. S., Grzywacz, J. G., & Zivnuska, S. (2009). Is work—family balance more than conflict and enrichment? *Human Relations, 62*(10), 1459–1486.

Clayton, S., Litchfield, C., & Geller, E. S. (2013). Psychological science, conservation, and environmental sustainability. *Frontiers in Ecology and the Environment, 11*, 377–382. https://doi.org/10.1890/120351

Cummins, R. A. (2005). The domains of life satisfaction: An attempt to order chaos. In *Citation classics from social indicators research* (pp. 559–584). Dordrecht: Springer.

Diener, E., Suh, E. M., Lucas, R. E., & Smith, H. L. (1999). Subjective well-being: Three decades of progress. *Psychological Bulletin, 125*(2), 276.

Duke, M. P. (1994). Chaos theory and psychology: Seven propositions. *Genetic, Social, and General Psychology Monographs, 120*(3), 267–286.

Duval, S., & Wicklund, R. A. (1972). *A theory of objective self-awareness*. New York: Academic Press.

Feldman, F. (2008). Whole life satisfaction concepts of happiness. *Theoria, 74*(3), 219–238.

Fitzgerald, R. (2016). *Human needs and politics*. Amsterdam: Elsevier.

Ho, A. (2008). The individualist model of autonomy and the challenge of disability. *Journal of Bioethical Inquiry, 5*(2), 193–207.

Kofodimos, J. R. (1993). *Balancing act*. San Francisco, CA: Jossey-Bass.

Lehman, B. J., David, D. M., & Gruber, J. A. (2017). Rethinking the biopsychosocial model of health: Understanding health as a dynamic system. *Social and Personality Psychology Compass, 11*(8), e12328.

Loewe, N., Bagherzadeh, M., Araya-Castillo, L., Thieme, C., & Batista-Foguet, J. M. (2014). Life domain satisfactions as predictors of overall life satisfaction among workers: Evidence from Chile. *Social Indicators Research, 118*(1), 71–86.

Matuska, K., Bass, J., & Schmitt, J. S. (2013). Life balance and perceived stress: Predictors and demographic profile. *OTJR: Occupation, Participation and Health, 33*(3), 146–158.

Robinson, S., & Notara, D. (2015). Building belonging and connection for children with disability and their families: A co-designed research and community development project in a regional community. *Community Development Journal, 50*(4), 724–741.

Rotter, J. B. (1990). Internal versus external control of reinforcement: A case history of a variable. *American Psychologist, 45*(4), 489.

Rotter, J. B. (1966). Generalized expectancies for internal versus external control of reinforcement. *Psychological Monographs: General and Applied, 80*(1), 1–28. https://doi.org/10.1037/h0092976.

Skar, P. (2004). Chaos and self-organization: Emergent patterns at critical life transitions. *Journal of Analytical Psychology, 49*(2), 243–262.

Stephens, L., Ruddick, S., & McKeever, P. (2015). Disability and Deleuze: An exploration of becoming and embodiment in children's everyday environments. *Body & Society, 21*(2), 194–220.

Suikkanen, J. (2011). An improved whole life satisfaction theory of happiness. *International Journal of Wellbeing, 1.* https://doi.org/10.5502/ijw.v1i1.6

Weiner, B. (1972). Attribution theory, achievement motivation, and the educational process. *Review of Educational Research, 42*(2), 203–215.

WHO. https://www.who.int/health-topics/health-promotion#tab=tab_1, accessed Feb 2022.

WHO. (2021). https://www.who.int/news-room/events/detail/2021/12/13/default-calendar/save-the-date---10th-global-conference-on-health-promotion-health-promotion-for-wellbeing-equity-and-sustainable-development, accessed Feb 2022.

Wilcock, A. A. (2007). Occupation and health: Are they one and the same? *Journal of Occupational Science, 14*(1), 3–8.

Yazdani, F., & Bonsaksen, T. (2017). Introduction to the model of occupational wholeness. *ErgoScience, 12*(1), 32-–36.

Yazdani, F., Roberts, D., Yazdani, N., & Rassafiani, M. (2016). Occupational balance: A study of the sociocultural perspective of Iranian occupational therapists: Équilibre occupationnel: Étude sur la perspective socioculturelle des ergothérapeutes iraniens. *Canadian Journal of Occupational Therapy, 83*(1), 53–62.

Zimbardo, P. (1985). *Psychology and life* (11th ed.). Northbrook, IL: Scott, Foresman, 653p.

2 The Model of Occupational Wholeness

Farzaneh Yazdani and Niayesh Fekri

Box 2.1 Chapter aims

This chapter will cover the definitions of the *MOW* components: *Occupational Wholeness, Being, Belonging, Becoming, Doings* and *Context*. This chapter also includes the relationship between components: *Being-Doings, Belonging-Doings, Becoming-Doings*, the relationship between components: *Being-Belonging* and *Being-Becoming*, illustration of the *MOW* as *Actual* and *Ideal Triangles* and finally the principles of the *MOW*.

The *Model of Occupational Wholeness (MOW)* is an aid for helpers (healthcare professionals in a helping capacity) to facilitate *Change* in a helpee (an individual who seeks help from a healthcare professional) towards better *Satisfaction* with themselves and their life, improve their *Well Being* and overall sense of integrity, contentment and *Wholeness*. Based on the *MOW*, human beings have not only the survival *Need* of existence but also the *Need* to live which is called a sense of *Being*. The *Need* for existing moves beyond an individual's *'Self'* to be part of something bigger than themself and that is called a sense of *Belonging*. Where the *Need* for existing extends further towards the future, it is considered as a sense of *Becoming*. All of these *Needs* are met through *Doings*. The *MOW* explains how the relationships between the above components contribute to the formation of a sense of *Wholeness* through *Doings*. An individual *Feels* well integrated and *Whole* if there is a positively *Meaningful* combination of *Doings* that help *Satisfy* their *Being, Belonging* and *Becoming (3Bs)*. These aspects of a person are illustrated in the *Hypothetical Triangle of Occupational Wholeness* (see Figure 2.1), the three vertices of which are *Being, Belonging* and *Becoming*. *Doings* are the central point of this *Triangle* that link the three vertices together. Occupation refers to *Doings* that act as a means to voluntarily and deliberately occupy time and space within a *Context*. Voluntary action in this context, and in connection with the definition of *Doings* provided above, and occupation mean the doer has *Control* over what they *Do/Not Do* through their brain system even if they have been forced externally. For instance, even when an external factor such as a particular law *Obliges* a person to *Do/Not Do* something, the act of *Doing* itself is under the person's *Control* and *Planned* by the motor cortex, thus *Doing* in this sense is not reflexive. The word *Control* should be carefully considered especially in relation to *Intention*. For example, a person with a neurological condition with tremor may have no *Control* over

DOI: 10.4324/9781003034759-2

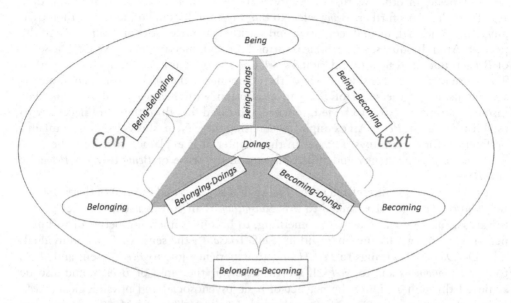

Figure 2.1 The Hypothetical Triangle of Occupational Wholeness

the movement itself but if they *Intend* to raise their arm and pick up something, their act, even if awkward, is still considered as *Doing*.

Similar to other *Health* and *Well Being* Models, the *MOW* consists of concepts that identify the fundamental assumptions of the model. The relationships between these concepts form the thinking process that is necessary in analysing and synthesizing the phenomena that are addressed by this model of *Occupational Wholeness (OW)*. In this section, each concept is explained individually; then the core concepts are explicated in relation to each other and also in connection to *Health* and *Well Being*.

Components of the sense of Occupational Wholeness (OW)

Below, the components of *OW* and the relationships between them are explained:

Being

Similar to Wilcock's definition of *Being*, the *MOW* conceptualizes the sense of *Being* as the human *Need* for a space just to '*Be*'. The *MOW* also adheres to the concept of *Being* introduced by Del Fabro Smith et al. (2011) which refers to the sense of *Being* as the way people understand themselves to *Be*, at present. An individual's *Being* evolves from the meeting of a survival, existing and living level to *Becoming*. In the very early stages of child development, alongside the basic physiological *Needs* for survival, the basic psychological *Needs* for *Autonomy*, competence and affiliation begin to take place (Vansteenkiste et al., 2020). An individual's *Being* developmentally extends towards *Belonging* and *Becoming*. There are pre-existing building blocks that act as predetermining factors for an individual's sense of *Being*. There is also impact of an individual's *Contexts* on further shaping and developing their sense of *Being*. Therefore, the interaction of an individual with their *Context*, explicitly and implicitly, influences their sense of *Being*, in other words, the individual's perception of themselves and who they are. To explain this further, *Being* refers to the way an individual understands their own physical, emotional, mental, cognitive and spiritual characteristics and *Capacities* in the present. An individual sense of *Being* is formed through meeting *Being Needs*. The sense of *Being* is not equivalent to individual's *Self* or sense of identity, although they overlap. The sense of *Being* is considered one of the components of *Self*. The other components are extensions of the sense of *Being* in association with *Belonging* and *Becoming*. For instance, an infant *Needs* to be fed, touched and cared for, all of these are necessary to establish a sense of *Being*. An example of exercising these *Needs* shows itself in an infant's preferences for certain toys. Further in this chapter, it is explained that how the *Need* for *Autonomy*, competency and affiliation expand the sense of *Being* towards *Belonging* and *Becoming*.

A sense of *Being* is also related to the *Feeling* of *Satisfaction* and the aim of that is intrinsic. A good *Feeling* that is linked to this *Satisfaction* is an end in itself. It is not geared towards a future goal, to achieve something, to become something better or to link a person with others. Its aim ends within itself. To *Satisfy* the sense of *Being*, individuals may *Do/Do Not Do* things to *Feel Happy*, to experience joy, to *Feel* present and alive, to *Feel Autonomous* and to *Feel* self-worth. *Satisfying* the sense of *Being* could also be achieved through avoiding the neglect of basic psychosocial and physiological *Needs*. Individuals shape their sense of *Being* through *Choice-Making* and *Meaning-Making* and by *Reflecting* on their *Doings*. Where an individual becomes directed towards discovering their *Capacity* which embraces what they can achieve, how they can grow, with whom they *Choose* to *Connect* and where and when they might go, their sense of *Being* extends to *Becoming and Belonging*.

Belonging

Belonging is an extension of *Being* that develops the person's sense of expansion of their *Being* through *Relationships* with others and affiliations with places, objects and concepts. The *MOW* agrees with Rogers (1951) in considering *Belonging* as a subjective experience and is about people's desire for *Connection* with others and to meet the *Need* for positive regard. The sense of *Belonging* is a subjective experience that does not necessarily depend on physical proximity or sharing space with others (Allen, 2020; Yazdani et al., 2021).

There are several ways in which an individual's sense of *Belonging* is formed. This can be through *Togetherness*, *Relatedness* and *Connectedness* with people, places, time, concepts and objects. It can be argued that the sense of *Belonging* begins to form when the foetus is in the womb. After birth, new-borns start a process of separation in order to develop their own self as a *Being*, although people may never *Feel* completely separated as an individual and left solely alone to meet their own *Needs*. People may go through this process of *Belonging/Separation* to different extents. In spite of the extent of this separation, a sense of *Belonging* re-emerges after an individual forms some level of *Selfhood*.

In the *MOW*, the sense of *Belonging* is not purely limited to social *Belonging* in relation to other people. The sense of *Belonging* extends to places, time, objects and concepts, too. It is important to consider that while a sense of *Belonging* is a *Motivator* for social participation, it is not equivalent to social participation. People may participate in a social activity without a sense of *Belonging* to the social group in which that activity is taking place. They may be participating due to *Obligations* or requirements of another life situation. For instance, a team manager may have *Expectations* of their team member attendance at a social event. However, in this *Context*, some members of the team may *Feel Related* to what is 'Done' at such a social event and indeed participate without *Relating* to the other team members. Within this group of attendees, there might be some who meet at least some of their *Belonging Needs* by being *Together* with their team members but may stay isolated even among others at that social event. Social *Belonging Needs* must be reciprocal to ensure *Satisfaction*; however, this is not the case for the sense of *Belonging* when *Related* to places, time, objects or concepts. The sense of *Belonging* to places, time, objects or concepts are strong aspects of people's identity which are powerfully related to subjective experiences of *Satisfaction* and deeply associated with their *Feelings* and *Emotions*.

In certain cases, there are external pressures which push a person to *Feel Belonging* towards a certain group, place or concept. These external pressures can be manifested in several ways, such as assumptions or *Expectations* made by others. *Dissatisfaction* may arise from a situation in which there is a *Discrepancy* or *Disharmony* between a person's sense of *Being* or *Becoming* and what they *Feel* the pressure to *Belong* to. The *Dissatisfaction* that may arise in the person *Feeling* that they ought to *Feel a sense of Belonging* to a certain group or place (sometimes/often) contrasts with the reality that they have a distinct sense of *Not Belonging*. However, *Dissatisfaction* can also be due to being externally categorized by others to be part of something that the person themself *Feels* has no positive *Meaning* in being *Connected* to. As a sense of *Belonging* is deeply associated with our sense of *Being*, managing the related conflicts is a complex process that provokes deep *Emotional* responses.

Not Belonging

Sense of *Not Belonging* may be experienced in two circumstances. The sense of *Not Belonging* may manifest itself in two main ways. One is related to an active attempt by a person to distance themself from a category which they *Feel* does not define them, and the other is more to do with external factors which prohibit the development of a sense of *Belonging*. An example of the former is when a person is assumed to hold certain ideological beliefs based on the way they look. For instance, a person who is from Southwest Asia who is assumed to be of Muslim faith may *Feel* no significant sense of *Belonging* to others within the Muslim community. However, over time, the assumption that some people may hold of the person makes them *Feel* excluded from other things in life that they may enjoy. This person may go out of their way to explain and show that they are not part of the Muslim community. For example, in the month of Ramadan that people of Muslim faith fast, this person may *Feel* the *Need* to make clear that others can invite them for coffee or food as they are not fasting. In this case, the person is practising their sense of *Not Belonging*. In cases where this external categorization is based on a prejudiced negative assumption about the person, the person's sense of *Not Belonging* may be stronger and more negative.

The other way in which a sense of *Not Belonging* can develop is when someone *Feels* excluded from a group, place or concept, which they *Want* to *Belong* to yet are prohibited from doing so based on other factors. Here, the sense of *Belonging* is internal, yet the external factors dominate and turn the person's sense of *Belonging* into *Not Belonging*. In the example above, the same issue is occurring in which the externally *Attributed* sense of *Belonging* does not match the internal one; however, in this case, it is the other way around. The person *Wants* to *Feel Belonging*, yet they are not externally included in this by others or their environment. Take, for example, a person who has spent considerable time perfecting their ability in playing classical music. Music is the passion of this person's life, and they have looked forward to making *Connections* with people who have similar interests. However, after years of hard work to get into a prestigious institution, they are faced with new challenges which hinder their sense of *Belonging*. Their own experiences, of coming from a lower socio-economic background and being a third-generation immigrant, *Meant* that they were socially excluded by others. Even though this person has music in common with those around them, they lack a sense of *Belonging* due to significant cultural differences. The sense of 'othering', as Jensen (2011) calls it, results in the person developing a sense of *Not Belonging* in spite of their desire to *Belong*.

Belonging levels: Togetherness, Relatedness and Connectedness

A sense of *Belonging* consists of various elements such as sharing, identification, similarities, closeness and trust. It is possible for an individual to *Attribute* positive or negative *Emotional Value* to their sense of *Belonging* in relation to a specific person, a group of people, a particular time or era, ideas and concepts or objects. A sense of *Belonging* is formed in three different layers: *Togetherness, Relatedness* and *Connectedness*. These three layers are hierarchically related to each other based on their *Value* and *Meaningfulness* for the individual. From *Togetherness* to *Relatedness* and finally *Connectedness*.

To be *Together* with others means sharing space, events and activities. Being *Together* could simply involve completing a task individually while sharing time and space with others such as sitting an examination. It can also include shared activities among a group of people, for example, playing football/hill walking/attending evening classes. While the link between individuals may be loose, there is still a level of *Belonging* that leads a person to be present in the given place and share time with others. Participating in an event and responding to its requirements within a group of people could be considered as *Togetherness*. Individuals may be part of a group yet not *Feel Connected* to the group or the people in it. *Togetherness* is a degree of the sense of *Belonging* that is defined by a superficial similarity with others, in one or more aspects of one's personal or *Contextual* characteristics, that has little *Value* or positive significance to a person.

Relatedness is one level deeper in shaping a sense of *Belonging*. This is when individuals have relations with one another, whether through kinship, professional or vocational setting or faith. For instance, at an international conference, participants may try to find people whom they *Feel* related. While some participants may try to find people from their own university or country, others may look for someone with similar profession or expertise.

Connectedness is one step deeper than *Relatedness*; it requires a deeper *Feeling* that goes beyond having something in common with others. To *Feel* a *Connection* to someone or something is to *Feel* a type of closeness. In relation to *Connectedness* with others, trust, mutual understanding and *Feeling* are valued elements that become more central. People may *Feel Related* to their siblings based on being raised in the same household, under the same faith and sharing similar memories. However, a person may *Feel* a stronger sense of *Connectedness* to one or other of their siblings based on a shared understanding of faith, a shared passion for creativity or a shared respect for each other's goals.

Reciprocity of *Feeling* which indexes a sense of *Belonging* between people may be present, but it is not essential for *Satisfying* the individual's sense of *Belonging*. However, more often than not, people's sense of *Belonging* develops in connection with some level of reciprocity. It is more common for non-reciprocal kinds of *Belonging* to be present when it is to do with *Belonging* to places, time, objects or concepts.

Becoming

Becoming develops as an extension of *Being* when humans' *Need* for exercising *Autonomy* and competence is linked to the future. *Becoming* is the dynamic process that moves humans beyond the present (Hitch et al., 2014). In other words, *Becoming* encompasses everything that ties a person to their future such as their hopes, aspirations and *Plans*. *Becoming* usually represents *Change*; however, it can also refer to the prevention of moving backwards or as Van Huet (2011) puts it: managing and maintaining. People may *Plan* to nurture their *Becoming* based on what they *Think* about their own capacities or interests that they have realized as part of their journey from *Being* to *Becoming*. People also develop an understanding of what their *Context* either *Expects* or *Demands* of them, and this influences their *Choice-Making* in relation to what they *Do/Not Do* to shape their *Becoming*. A sense of *Control* and *Attainment* that starts as a *Need* for *Being* is exercised towards *Becoming*. To succeed in *Satisfying* one's *Becoming Needs*, it is necessary for individuals to understand their own *Capacities* and the influence of *Contextual Factors* on their *Doings*, *Choice-Making* and *Meaning-Making*. In other words, a sense of *Becoming* is linked to the relationship between an individual and who or what they *Feel* they *Belong* to. In some cases, *Satisfying* the *Expectations* placed on an individual by their families, social circles or society at large is the most significant guiding factor for their sense of *Becoming*. In such cases, personal interests and capacities are less determinant factors in shaping the sense of *Becoming*.

It is important to note that *Becoming* is not always about moving forward, sustaining an individual's circumstances and maintaining their state of *Being* is considered as *Becoming,* too. This kind of *Becoming* can particularly be seen when people have reached a relatively *Satisfying* state of their life which they would like to maintain. Additionally, while some people prefer to maintain a *Satisfactory* situation, others may start looking for new challenges.

Doing/Not Doing (Doings)

Doing/Not Doing (Doings) are at the core of the *MOW.* It is through both categories of *Doings* that the sense of *Being, Belonging* and *Becoming* is developed. Based on the *MOW,* both *Doing* and *Not Doing* are required to be *Intentional*. The *Intentional* form of *Doing*, such as taking a shower, attending an event or applying for a job, contributes to meeting the *Needs* of *Being, Belonging* and *Becoming*. The *Intentional Not Doing* such as not going to specific places, not participating in certain activities and not leading a particular lifestyle is a *Planned Not Doing* that involves *Choice-Making* and *Meaning-Making*.

Earlier in this chapter, it was stated that part of our *Being* is predetermined. As the senses of *Belonging* and *Becoming* are developed as extensions of *Being*, to some extent, they are influenced by those pre-existing factors, as well. Further development of *Being* and consequently *Belonging* and *Becoming* occurs as a result of an individual's *Doings*. To claim that *Doings* are the means for the formation and development of the *3Bs (Being, Belonging and Becoming)* indicates the necessity of a clear definition of *Doings* and the extent to which human action comes under *Doings*. For instance, it is necessary to decide whether the implicit aspects of *Doing* should include *Intention* and *Planning*, which happen internally, or whether as Cutchin et al. (2008) state, *Doing* refers to actions which are clearly physical, not sedentary or mental, *Doings*. In the *MOW*, *Doings* are those which are presented externally, they are actions that take place externally as opposed to thought or imagination that happen internally. *Doings* are not the implicit processes behind actions. An example of imaginary action is when individuals imagine themselves playing football, or driving, and the like. These imaginations are different from what happens in the brain system that guides the external presentation of actions. In a way, *Doings* have implicit and subjective representation as well as explicit actions that take place outside of a person and are observable. There are times when due to physical impairments and consequent limitations, *Doings* may fit into an imaginary *Doing*. For instance, Ashley, a child with cerebral palsy with interest in playing football in the playground, plays a football game using a play station and imagines himself as one of the football players. He told others that he plays football. To him this is what he *Does*. There is a combination of explicit *Doing* that is using the play equipment and imaginary *Doing*. Therefore, the *MOW* considers that as a form of *Doing* that is called imaginary *Doing* as it has the element of intention and it is not merely dreaming about an action or idea. The next question is whether *Doings* cover involuntary human actions such as breathing, seeing and hearing. The answer is no. According to the *MOW*, *Doings* are required to be *Voluntary* (opposed to reflexive) and *Intentional*. The *Intention* an individual has for *Not Doing* is equally a means for meeting the *Needs* of *Being, Belonging* and *Becoming*.

Another question is related to the *Purpose* and *Meaning Assigned* to *Doings*. Is it necessary for *Doings* to have an *Intentional Purpose* and *Meaning* in order to be considered as a means of meeting the *Needs* for *Being, Belonging* and *Becoming*. There are two aspects to be considered in addressing *Doings* as a *Purposeful* or *Meaningful* action. *Purpose* is necessary for *Doings*, although, as Hitch et al. (2014) pose, "whose *Purpose*" needs to be considered for *Doing*: that of the individual themself or that of the observant? The *MOW* response is that regardless of whether *Purpose* is identified by the doer or by someone external to them, *Purpose* is necessary for human acts to be considered as human *Doings*. People may have different perspectives on the *Purpose* of a particular *Doing*. Most *Doings* have a *Purpose* by nature. For example, a person with dementia tends to their *Need* for food by eating. They may *Feel* confused about the *Purpose* of this action, to the extent that they may not be able to link their *Need* and their actions together. However, the act of eating in its nature has a *Purpose*. In other words, it does not matter what an individual's cognitive *Capacity* permits and whether it allows making the connection between the *Doings* and their *Purpose*. This person has the *Intention* to *Do* and their act of eating is not a reflexive act even though they may not have insight about the outcome of this action.

Meaningfulness, though, is another issue for discussion. *Meaningfulness* is the positive or negative *Emotional Value* that is *Assigned* to something. While it is more common to see the word *Meaningful* used in occupational science and psychology as something that refers to a positive *Value* and therefore as a driver for *Doings* (Hasselkus, 2011; Ikiugu & Pollard, 2015), the *MOW* puts emphasis on the different *Values Attributed* to the *Meaning* of a concept or action. According to the *MOW*, *Meaningfulness* may signify a positive or negative *Value* and both of these may *Motivate* or *Demotivate Doings*.

In this chapter, seven scenarios are presented to help with understanding the relationships between *Meaning, Purpose* and *Doings* and link between different components of the *MOW*. Scenario 2.1 demonstrates *Assigning* a negative *Meaning, Attributing* adverse *Value* and *Motivation* for *Not Doing*. Scenario 2.2 illustrates the link between the *Assignment* of a negative *Meaning* and the *Demotivating* role it plays for *Doings*. Scenario 2.3 draws a comparison between the *Purpose* versus *Meaning Assigned to Doings*. Scenario 2.4 shows the link between *Being* and *Becoming* and Scenario 2.5 the link between *Becoming* and *Belonging*. Scenario 2.6 and 2.7 show some examples of *Contextual Factors*, and Scenario 2.8 demonstrates *Incongruence* between the *Actual* and *Ideal Triangles*. 2.9 explains some of the *MOW* principles in understanding a helpee's narrative. These scenarios are based on real stories with pseudonyms.

Scenario 2.1

Assigning negative Meaning

Ben, who is 25 years old, believes that a young man of his age should practise abstinence and considers sexual relationships before marriage unacceptable. Here, the *Meaning Assigned* to intimate relationships before marriage is negative which *Motivates* Ben towards *Not Doing*. This negative *Assignment* of *Meaning* to intimate relationships before marriage has turned into a strong *Motivation* for him to *Do* things that prepare him for married life such as saving money and getting a secure job. It can be argued that this is a positive *Meaning Assigned* to married lifestyle that meets his *Need* for a sexual relationship that counts as a *Motivator*. While this can be true, looking into this scenario more deeply and unfolding Ben's story further it becomes clear that if what he *Values* is not about building family life at this stage of Ben's life that *Motivates* him, it is in fact the avoidance of an action that has significant negative *Meaning* that *Motivates* him. This brief example indicates the significance of the impact that a negative *Meaning* for *Doing* and its link to *Values Attributed* to that can have on an individual's *Motivation* for action that may be stronger than the positive outcome of an action.

There are acts that by their nature may be considered as negative or positive, while there are other *Doings* that only in relation to their consequent impact on an individual's sense of *Being*, *Belonging* and *Becoming* are considered as negative or positive. The *Meaning-Making* that underpins *Doings* is related to what is considered to be the impact of *Doings* on the sense of *Being*, *Belonging* and *Becoming*.

Scenario 2.2

Significantly negative Meaning and Demotivation

Maria has hemiplegia after her stroke. She is refusing to walk, as she *Feels* that her pathological walking pattern is embarrassing. She is not *Motivated* to practise gait exercises as she finds these useless because they would not help her to walk normally. The word *useless* here indicates the *Meaning* that Maria *Assigns* to these exercises which she finds significantly negative and a waste of time. So, gait exercise has a significant negative *Meaning* that *Demotivated* Maria's commitment to *Doing* them.

Maria's scenario raises a question as to whether being positively *Meaningful* is necessary for what a person does or does not *Do* in order to call it *Doings*? The answer is, No. But is it necessary to consider the role that *Meaning-Making* plays in linking *Doings* to the sense of *Being*, *Belonging* and *Becoming*. The point is that *Doings* may have positive/negative *Meaning* and at times may have no *Meaning* for a person. Therefore, understanding the *Meaning* made or *Assigned* to *Doings* seems to be necessary in the way that *Doings* can meet the *Needs* for individuals' sense of *Being, Belong* and *Becoming*. The issue of *Meaning-Making* is an important and simultaneously complex aspect of the *MOW.*

An example to show the impact of considering a *Purpose* compared to *Assigning Meaning* to *Doings* and its *Motivating/Demotivating Value* can be seen in Scenario 2.3.

Scenario 2.3

Lia has insomnia and finds it extremely debilitating as he becomes restless and tired during the day. His helper has been discussing several options that Lia could try to see if they have an impact on his sleep. One of the options was to listen to meditative music an hour before bedtime. Lia considered this activity annoying but agreed to try it for the *Purpose* of facilitating his sleep. Later, he reported that it had no impact on his sleep and what mattered to him was not being unable to sleep but the negative consequences of the lack of sleep.

Here, the helper indicated to Lia that the annoying, or negative, *Meaning Assigned* to the suggested activity may have had a negative impact on the outcome. Therefore, even though Lia was *Doing* the act that was suggested and had a *Purpose*, the negative *Assignment* of *Meaning* to that may have influenced the effectiveness of what he was *Doing*.

Being–Belonging

Being a foetus in a mother's womb is the first innate *Connection* between an individual and others. Perhaps for babies growing out of a womb, a *Connection* that a foetus would have made with the mother is substituted by *Connection* to an equipment. Psychological theories hold that the very earliest stages of development for a child in establishing their *Selfhood* is to create boundaries between their own *Being* and the mother's breast or any equivalent means of feeding (Ashbach & Schermer, 2005). It appears that forming a sense of *Being* is initiated by a separation followed by establishing a connection again. This matter makes the relationship between the sense of *Being* and the sense of *Belonging* a complex phenomenon. While having a distinct sense of *Being* is essential for human development, an individual *Being* finds its *Meaning* in relation to others: people, places, objects, living creatures, time and events. Later in this chapter, it is discussed how an individual's *Contexts* have an impact on the formation of their sense of *Being* and how the sense of *Being*, in turn, influences an individual's *Connections* and *Relationships*.

Being–Becoming

Taking action from actual *Being* towards potentials is the basis for the development of *Being* towards *Becoming*. When an individual *Plans* and commits to turning their current characteristics and *Capacities* to what and how they *Think* they can *Be*, the sense of *Being* extends to the sense of *Becoming*. There are several factors contributing to the extension of *Being* to *Becoming* and ensuring the outcome of the *Change* that an individual is *Predicting*. What an individual *Expects* to *Become* is based on their perceived sense of *Being*. The impact of the sense of *Being* on a person's *Becoming* is a two-way process. The outcome of what an individual has *Planned* to achieve influences their sense of *Being* as well. Here is a short scenario as an example to explain the link between *Being* and *Becoming*.

Scenario 2.4

James's sense of *Being* at present indicates his perception of his *Capacity* for *Becoming* a singer. He sees the right talent in himself, therefore he hopes and *Plans* to *Become* a successful singer in two years after attending classes, learning the skills required and getting practice. Therefore, what James sees himself as at present time is a person who is interested in singing and has the potential to *Become* a professional/an experienced singer. To move from his *Being* to *Becoming*, James commits himself to a *Plan*. In two years' time when he is *Satisfied* as a singer, his sense of *Being Changes* from that of potential singer to an actual singer.

Becoming–Belonging

The relationship between *Belonging* and *Becoming* is complicated because *Belonging* also overlaps with individuals' *Context*. An individual's *Values* are interconnected with whom and what they *Feel* they *Belong* or don't *Belong*. *Planning* for the future could be related to people, ideas or places that individuals *Want* to be part of and have a sense of *Belonging* to. The following scenario demonstrates an example of the sense of *Belonging* in relation to *Becoming*.

Scenario 2.5

Sina is a high-school student *Planning* to study sport rehabilitation in further education. His interest in the subject is influenced by his positive *Values* towards being part of the athletic community. However, for Sina to study sport rehabilitation, he needs to move out of his hometown as the course is not offered locally. Sina's sense of *Belonging* is currently very *Connected* to his family and friends at home. Because of this, Sina's sense of *Becoming*, based on pursuit of his studies, and his sense of *Belonging*, which relies on close ties to family and friends, seem to be at odds with each other. Although pursuing his sense of *Becoming* is still associated with his sense of *Belonging*, Sina also *Values* being a part of the occupational community of sports rehabilitators.

Sense of Occupational Wholeness

A sense of *Wholeness* portrays the interactions between an individual's *Being*, *Belonging* and *Becoming* and their *Context*. *Doings* is the means of forming these complex interactions. According to the *MOW*, *Doing/Not Doing* is through *Intentional* occupying of time and space, and as such, it is called occupation. The concept of *Occupational Wholeness* refers to people's sense of *Being Whole* through their *Doings*.

Context

The *MOW* considers time and space as key factors in the surroundings of an individual. The concept of time is considered in two ways: time in relation to the continuum of an individual's life and time in the continuum of the historical moment in which they are situated at local, national and global levels.

Being, Belonging, Becoming and Doings are all situated within the *Context* of the individual's surroundings. What weaves all these components together is *Doings*, while the surroundings and *Contextual Factors* frame an individual's multi-layered sense of *Predicting*,

Expecting, Demanding, Encouraging, Facilitating, Supporting, Restricting, Inhibiting, Blocking and *Opposing* (see Table 2.1).

Space also may refer to an individual's relative position in their family, community or society. Here, the definition of community is based on a variety of elements, such as geography, ideology and interests (James et al., 2012). An individual's surroundings contribute hugely to the formation and development of the sense of *Being, Belonging* and *Becoming.* The impact of *Context* is evident even in a culture in which *Being* is portrayed as an individualistic sense of *Self* rather than the collective view of *Self* in relation to others (Lyons et al., 2002). For instance, people's sense of *Being* as independent individuals is associated with what independence means in the society that people live in. In many Western societies, people would consider independence in connection with finance, exercising *Choice* and making decisions. For instance, a 24-year-old woman may demonstrate her independence by making a decision to get married and support herself to provide the finances for the wedding. So, the sense of *Being* that has been formed around independence is still based on the definition of independence in her society. In a collective society, a woman of the same age may still form a sense of independence whilst the term independence may have a different definition. In the latter case, consulting parents and relying on their financial support for a wedding does not contradict the notion of *Being* independent as the societal assumption is that young people are required to be supported financially at the beginning of their adult life, and it is deemed to be the parents' responsibility to support this. Therefore, within this *Context,* independence is exercised through the person's *Choice* of partner, but does not include financial independence from their family. Apart from differences in the dimensions of independence that may differ based on individual and societal *Values*, there are also *Contexts* in which the independence of young people in relation to establishing a new life, completely separate from their parents, has no *Meaning* or *Value.* Therefore, an individual's sense of *Being* in such a *Context* is massively integrated with their sense of *Belonging.* Elements of people's surroundings, therefore, are diverse and their influential power in forming and developing their sense of *Being, Belonging* and *Becoming* varies. The *Meaning* of *Doings* as well as the *Expected* impact of *Doings* on an individual's sense of *Being, Belonging* and *Becoming* is largely dependent on the *Expectations, Demands* or support of *Contextual Factors.* Scenario 2.6 illustrates the role community *Values* play in a person's sense of *Being, Belonging* and *Becoming.*

Scenario 2.6

Ayodele, a young Australian man, has recently gone through an operation to amputate both his arms. He is struggling with his Sense of *Being, Becoming* and *Belonging* and is referred to a helper to discuss his new situation that has hugely impacted his *Doings.* Understanding Ayodele's sense of *Being, Belonging and Becoming* prior to his accident is essential in helping him to manage his current situation and improve his *Well Being.*

Since Ayodele was a little boy, similar to most boys in his community, he avidly attended swimming classes every week. His concept of *Being* was very much associated with his regular swimming, *Being* a swimmer and *Being* a young athlete who led a *Healthy* lifestyle. Swimming provided him with an *Opportunity* to connect with several groups of people. Ayodele's hobbies with his friendship group all revolved around swimming. His volunteering work, to help elderly people in the swimming pool, was considered a respectful activity, particularly for a young man of his age. In his small town, people were always praising him for his success in swimming competitions and supporting his dream to represent his town at national level. Ayodele's scenario represents the extent of influence that community *Values* had on his sense of *Being, Belonging* and *Becoming*.

The above example demonstrates the impact of geography and the significance of swimming within the culture of the community. It is clear that Ayodele's community views the ability to swim an essential skill. Ayodele has internalized this *Value* as part of his *Being* and also developed his sense of *Belonging* and *Becoming* around it. In the interaction between his *Being* and *Becoming*, he has expanded the potential of his love of swimming to achieve acknowledgement for his swimming skills which has also strengthened his *Connections* with local community groups. The community validation and respect for what Ayodele *Does* strengthens his sense of *Being* in relation to swimming.

Every individual's sense of *Being, Belonging* and *Becoming* is framed by their *Contexts* through *Expecting, Demanding, Encouraging, Facilitating, Supporting, Restricting, Blocking, Opposing* their *Doings*. Table 2.1 draws on Ayodele's scenario to illustrate the roles that *Context* plays in a person's *Doings*.

Ayodele's story illustrates how his *Context* has framed his sense of *Being, Belonging* and *Becoming* through his *Doings*. The easy access to swimming pools and beaches in his town *Facilitates* his *Doings*. Furthermore, Ayodele's family provide *Support* through

Table 2.1 Contextual roles, definition and examples

Role	Definition	Example shows how these factors would have been related to Ayodele's scenario
Expecting	Believing about something that influences *Doings*	The family and community *Expect* Ayodele to achieve a certain level of skills in swimming
Demanding	Insisting or requiring certain *Doings*	The local authorities *Demanded* Ayodele to attend school like other children when he was in school age
Encouraging	Instilling hope and confidence for *Doings*	Comments such as "That's a good idea, I am sure you can represent this town at national swimming competitions" from members of community represents *Encouragement*
Facilitating	Make *Doings* easier	A local leisure club gives Ayolede a free access to their swimming pool for practising and helping elderly people
Supporting	Bearing part of all of the weight to make *Doings* happen	Ayoledel's parent Support him by paying for the swimming classes, swimming gear and equipment
Restricting	Putting a limit on, commanding *Doings*	Ayolede could not attend some of the competitions he was invited to due to limited affordable transportation to the venue
Blocking	Preventing *Doings*	Ayodele would have experienced *Blocking* if there was no beach or swimming pool that he could have access
Opposing	Causing conflict in *Doings* or competing with *Doings*	This would happen if Ayodele's parent or teachers would have *Opposed* to his engagement with swimming

enrolling him in swimming classes and buying him the relevant equipment for attending swimming competitions. Ayodele's story does not show any *Demand* on him from either his family or society to be a swimmer. However, his achievements made him known to his community and gradually raised *Expectations* of him *Being* a successful athlete to make a name for his town. Ayodele takes this very seriously and hopes to make the people in his town proud. It's important to note that there is a difference between the actual presence of *Facilities,* level of *Support, Demand, Expectation* and Ayodele's perception of them. While parental praising of a child's performance may be perceived as strong support by one child, another may not perceive it in the same way. The issue of what the actual *Contextual Factors* are and how an individual perceives them is an important point of consideration when it comes to understanding people as helpees.

Contextual Factors can refer to geography, weather and natural resources like Ayodele's access to swimming or it can refer to the historical, political or ideological *Context* within which the individual is situated. Each one of these elements can provide or inhibit *Opportunities*. Below, in Scenario 2.7, another example of contributing *Contextual Factors* opens discussion about the role *Contextual Factors* play in people's *OW* and its components.

Scenario 2.7

Charlotta lives in a country that has recently *Changed* politically which is more restrictive in relation to women's presence and activities in society. Her family *Belongs* to a minority religious group whose rights are infringed upon frequently.

Being a member of a marginalized group that is not officially recognized by the government, Charlotta has grown up with a strong sense of her religious identity. The negative societal attitudes towards her religion have led to a strong association between her sense of *Being* and *Belonging* to her religious community. Charlotta was informed at a young age that she does not have the right to higher education in her country. The *Blocking* of *Opportunities* such as access to higher education amongst other universal rights such as the right to vote has hugely affected the development of her sense of *Being* in relation to her community group and not to her nationality. It is not strange that Charlotta hopes to live in a place that provides her with more *Opportunities* and *Plans* to migrate to another country that may *Support* her and *Facilitate Doings* that aid fulfilling her *Needs* in *Becoming* a nurse.

Triangle of Occupational Wholeness

The *MOW* is shaped as a *Triangle*, and the relationships between the components of the *OW* are presented via this *Triangle*. *Doings*, placed in the centre of the *Triangle*, is considered as an intermediate *Need* to ensure that the *Needs* of *Being, Belonging* and *Becoming* (placed at the three apexes) are met. Therefore, no matter who the person, there is always a *Hypothetical Triangle* based on these *Needs*. This is called the *Triangle of Human Occupational Wholeness*. The *Hypothetical Triangle* has equilateral sides to illustrate a *Congruent* and well-integrated person.

The core of the model is based on the concept of *OW* that refers to a sense of *Being* in one piece as a Whole. People *Feel* well integrated, content and *Whole* if they perceive a positive *Meaningful* combination of what they *Do/Not Do* in order to meet their *Needs* for the *3Bs*. A state of *Balance*, characterized by all three *Needs* being met to a sufficient extent, allows the person to experience a state of *OW*. To represent a *Satisfactory* situation, the word *Harmony* is used to explain the combination of positively *Meaningful* and significant *Doings* that form an individual's sense of *OW*.

The state of *OW* continuously shifts based on *Changes* in the sense of *Being, Belonging* and *Becoming*. Therefore, an individual is always moving towards or away from a sense of *OW* which is temporary and relative. This means that at different times and stages of people's lives, there can be states of *OW* and the lack thereof, and the individual's proximity to *OW* can oscillate.

The *MOW* introduces a *Triangle* that illustrates the relationship between its elements *Hypothetically*. Then, examples are provided to present potentially real situations. One *Triangle* refers to the relationship between the four elements in an *Actual* situation and the other illustrates an *Ideal* situation. The *Incongruence* between the two represents a *Gap. Congruence/Incongruence of the Actual and Ideal Triangles* are one of the determinants of potential *Satisfaction* or its lack that individual has with what they *Do/Not Do* and the way it helps them to *Feel* as a *Whole, Content* and may be *Happy*.

Each individual leads their life in a particular way that is called their *Actual* situation. The *Actual* situation refers to what people *Actually Do/Not Do* to meet their *Needs* for *Being, Belonging* and *Becoming*. The *Actual* situation, which is illustrated by the *Actual Triangle* (see Figure 2.2), refers to the present. However, each individual could have an *Ideal* situation for their life pattern that may or may not diverge from their *Actual* situation. The *Ideal* situation is represented by the *Ideal Triangle* (see Figure 2.2). The more *Congruence* between the two (*Actual* and *Ideal*) *Triangles*, the greater a person's *Life Satisfaction, Self-Fulfilment* and sense of *Wholeness*. However, *Congruence* does not necessarily mean that it is the best objective situation for the person in terms of their mental/physical *Health*. Examples illustrating the *Congruence* or *Incongruence* of *Actual* and *Ideal Triangles* are presented in the chapters that follow.

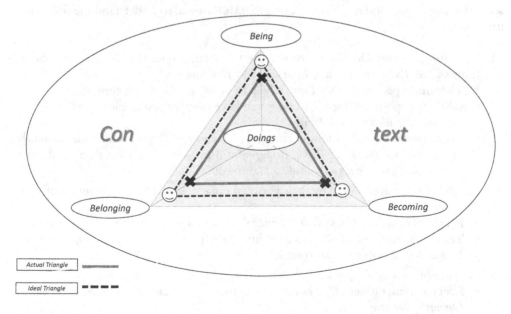

Figure 2.2 The Hypothetical Actual and Ideal Triangles

Scenario 2.7 below introduces extreme examples of *Incongruence* between Lotaria's *Actual* and *Ideal Triangle*.

Scenario 2.8

Lotaria is a teacher who spends most of her working day and free time in school. She *Feels* very anxious about her teaching and usually forgets to have her lunch as one of the most basic *Bing Need*. Lotaria's *Actual* situation reveals that she has little time for her own children and mostly attends to only their basic *Needs*, such as washing their clothes and cooking for them that makes her *Feel Unhappy* with her sense of *Belonging*. Lotaria has a playful nature and has always *Valued Being* a mother who spends a lot of time with her children. However, she is *Obliged* to work to provide for her family. She is frustrated by not meeting her *Belonging Needs*. She wishes that one day she can go back to the university and take her master degree in education.

Lotaria's scenario shows the *Incongruence* between her *Actual* and *Ideal Triangles*. Upon identifying the *Incongruence* in these two *Triangles*, the helper and Lotaria need to agree on their next action that is designing a *Tailored (Reality) Triangle* that is the aim of the *Change* they agree on. The *MOW* uses *Empowering* and *Enabling* strategies to aid these *Changes*. The *Triangles* and intervention strategies are explained in detail in other chapters.

Principles of the MOW

Helpers are required to adhere to the *MOW* principle, at all steps of the *MOW*-based intervention. Success in an *MOW*-based intervention depends on helpers' knowledge and skills of employing the *MOW* principles when in a helping position. These principles are introduced below, and throughout the book, they are expanded and used in scenarios where appropriate. Helpers using the *MOW* need to understand the following nine points.

1 The things people *Do/Not Do* contribute to meeting one, two or more combinations of the *3B Needs of Being, Belonging* and *Becoming*.
   • The things people *Do/Not Do* that help to meet one *Need* may contradict another.
   • *Choices* people make for their *Doings* can have positive and negative consequences for their *Health* and *Well Being*.
   • An exaggerated and/or long–term *Skewed Triangle* of *Doings*, which insufficiently meets all three *Needs* for *Being, Belonging* and *Becoming*, leads to a decreased sense of *OW* and can potentially lead to *Health* issues.
2 People's *Choices* are limited by their personal capacities and by the resources of their *Contexts*.
   • People may make a *Choice* to meet one *Need*, although this may overshadow others.
   • There are realities of life, such as human capacities, *Contextual Opportunities, Demands* and occupational complexities that limit human *Choices*.
3 People not only *Make Choices* but also make *Meanings* and *Assign* to them.
   • Everyone encounters *Contextual* and personal *Obligations* that restrict options, *Opportunities* and *Choices*.
   • Positive *Meaning-Making* of an *Obligation* is *Healthier* than not finding any *Meaning* in *Obligations* or considering them to be completely negative.

- People *Attribute* positive or negative *Values* to their *Doings* and the *Meaning* they *Assign* to those *Meanings*.
- Positive *Meaning-Making* and *Attribution* of positive *Value* to *Doings* contribute to a sense of *Self-Fulfilment*, *Life Satisfaction* and *Subjective Well Being*.

4 Occupational *Choices* and *Meaning-Making* are not only an individual but also a social matter.
- Positive subjective experiences of a situation can help to reduce the negative impact of some of the *Doings* in which people engage due to social *Obligations*.

5 *Congruence* between *Actual* and *Ideal Triangles*, their *Meaning* and *Attributions* of *Values* should be analysed and evaluated in both objective and subjective ways.
- Each individual has their own unique profile representing combinations of *Doings*.
- The level of *Incongruence Changes* throughout people's lives.
- A *Reality Triangle* should be *Planned* to help people to achieve the best possible *Congruence*.
- Long-term, *Skewed Triangles* can potentially impact on an individual's *Health* and *Well Being*
- The issues of time and stage of a person's life, along with the *Meaning* made and *Values Attributed* to a *Skewed Situation* and its duration, are significant in relation to the degree of effect it has on individual's life, *Health* and *Well Being*.
- While *Incongruence* between the *Actual* situation of a person's profile and the *Ideal* one is natural, a significant *Incongruence* that is intensive and long term could put a person's *Health* at risk.
- For an individual to *Feel* well integrated, contented and *Whole*, all their *Needs* have to be met to some extent.
- *Harmony* among *Doings* that serves *Being, Belonging* and *Becoming* is necessary for an individual's *Health* and *Well Being*.

6 The significance of *Self-Awareness*.
   OW might not be brought into helpee's consciousness automatically. In the *Context* of the subjective experience of *Health* and *Well Being*, it is necessary to make people aware of the link between what they *Do/Not Do* and how their *Doings* within their *Context* are associated with their *Needs* of *Being, Belonging* and *Becoming*. In other words, the sense of *OW* is achieved through the person's recognition of their *Doings* and the effects produced by them.

7 The aim of intervention is to raise *Self-Awareness* about individual's *Thinking, Feeling and Doings* in relation to their *Being, Belonging* and *Becoming* and their *Contextual Factors*. Through this, people may be able to make *Changes* towards meeting their *Needs* and approaching a sense of *Wholeness*. The '*Change*' is the intervention in the *MOW*.

8 *Changes* in one or more components of an individual's sense of *OW* impact the others and the overall sense of *OW*. While the outcome can be *Predicated* to some extent, it never can be absolute as there are always unseen factors or interactions of factors that would influence *Change* and consequently outcome.

9 If people have difficulty in making a positive *Meaning* and *Attributing* positive *Value* to their situation, they may become *Dissatisfied* with themselves and/or their lives. This may be when their *Doings* do not meet their *Needs* of *Being, Belonging* and *Becoming* or when these are not in *Harmony* with each other.

Scenario 2.9 explains some of the above *MOW* principles in understanding a helpee's narrative.

Scenario 2.9

Jagnu works 13 hours a day to bring in income for his family that includes his wife, three children and his elderly parent, as well as his younger brother with mental *Health* issues. His job pays him well but does nothing to *Satisfy* his ambitions. Jagnu loves singing and has always dreamed of *Being* a professional singer but the amount of time he spends on earning money does not leave him any *Opportunity* to pursue his ambition. He leads this *Dissatisfying* lifestyle as he *Feels* he has no other *Choice*. Jagnu's friend Antec is in a similar situation, but he *Feels* fine as he *Thinks* that taking care of his family is *Valuable* and does not mind postponing his ambition. Antec believes the good things he *Does* will bring good to him in the future, and being *Connected* to his family makes him *Feel* strong.

The above comparison between Jagnu and Antec shows the difference in perception and *Meaning* of the *Skewed Triangle* in what they *Do/Not Do* to meet their *Needs* for *Being, Belonging* and *Becoming*. Jagnu obviously cannot make a positive *Meaning, Feels* he has no *Choice*, sees himself as a victim and is *Unhappy* about it. In contrast, Antec accepts his situation as an *Obligation* but understands that he has responded to this *Obligation* by making a helpful *Meaning* and *Attributes* a positive *Value* to it. It appears that Antec is *Happier*, more *Satisfied* and *Feels* more content than Jagnu. In other words, a cognitive justification and *Reality* orientation towards Antec's life situation has helped, to some extent, to provide him with a more constructive experience. However, the impact of their *Skewed* lifestyles on them in the long term should not be denied.

Individuals *Feel* better, more content and *Satisfied* with their life when they *Feel* what they *Do/Not Do* works towards fulfilling their *Needs* of *Being* who they sense they are and can be (*Becoming*). The individuals who are more *Satisfied* with their lives also seem to be those who can *Do/Not Do* things that keep them *Connected* to something or somebody. However, there are also examples of people who go too far to keep their *Connection* and *Belonging* to other things, places or people and this leads to them neglecting themselves, who they are and what they *Want* to *Become*. Some of these individuals place ideological *Value* in other's *Happiness*, which helps them stay *Happier* and relatively more content with what they *Do/Not Do*. Some people may find their potential *Being* wasted in others' wills and have not loved themselves enough to invest in their own dreams. Jagnu and Antec highlight these differences.

Greatest *Life Satisfaction* can be seen among people who have a well-defined, positively *Meaningful* and integrated sense of *Being*. People who can explain their *Choices* and in connection with what they *Do/Not Do* and have *Awareness* about their *Choices* and *Responsibilities* are more likely *to Feel* content with themselves and their life.

The right combination of *Doings* to meet the *3Bs Needs* is not necessarily an equal amount of time and energy spent in meeting each one of the *OW* components. Some people with a *Skewed* occupational profile have a rationale for their *Choices* and accept the *Responsibility* for that. They also have explanations for and acceptance of their *Obligations*, which can help them agree to them more easily, even if it has a negative impact on their *Health*. Antec obviously finds working too hard exhausting, but within his belief system, serving his family is *Valued*. He *Thinks* his family's blessing will bring *Opportunities* in the future. He also *Thinks* the situation will *Change* when his children are grown and more independent. In addition, he complains about the long hours and his back pain due to it. He has hopes and therefore has some ideas as to how he can *Plan* for the future to cut down his hours. Antec said,

I know I cannot and I also believe I should not go on like that. No matter how much I *Feel* good about supporting my family and *Thinking* spiritually about this, I am *Aware* that in the long term this hard physical work will damage my *Health* and that is not going to help anyone....

The above scenarios show the significant role of *Making Choice*, in particular a well-informed *Choice,* and accepting *Reality* that, in turn, can help a more positive, subjective experience of the right combination of what is *Done/Not Done*.

Stages of life development and sense of Occupational Wholeness

People's sense of *Being, Belonging* and *Becoming* and resulting *OW* is fluid. While there are aspects of an individual's *Being, Belonging* and *Becoming* that take shape in the very early stages of life, these components constantly *Change* throughout an individual's life. The stage of an individual's life and their age are determining influential factors in the *Changes* that happen in these three *Needs* components and the overall sense of *OW*. In fact, the sense of *OW* is never fully achieved, but it is something that an individual moves towards in all stages of life. Paradoxically, in moving towards achieving *OW*, individuals may keep moving away from it.

For instance, while the basic physiological *Needs* exist throughout people's life, their contribution to a person's sense of *Being* differs in different ages and stages of an individual's life. An extreme example is the political activism of an individual whose *Doings* lead to incarceration and hunger strike. This example indicates an individual whose sense of *Being* has developed around a strong sense of *Becoming* and who stands by their

---

Box 2.2 Activities for learning and reflection

These activities are aimed at helping you to practise the concepts of the *MOW* and create *Actual* and *Ideal Triangles of OW*:

Activity 1.2

*   Give three examples of how you meet your own *Needs* for *Being, Belonging and Becoming*.

Activity 2.2

*   Create the *Actual Triangle* of your *3Bs of Doings*.
*   Create the *Ideal Triangle* of your *3Bs of Doings*.

Answer these questions to help you analyse your own *OW* situation:

*   Identify the *Incongruence* between your two *Actual* and *Ideal Triangles*.
*   What are the personal and *Contextual Factors* that contribute to any potential *Incongruence/Gap*?
*   How do you *Feel* about this *Incongruence/Gap*?

beliefs. Another example is a woman who is living in poverty and whose sense of *Being* is interwoven with her sense of *Belonging* to her children. In spite of the presence of basic *Needs* for survival, her sense of *Being* a mother informs her *Doings* towards taking care of her children. In turn her *Doings Empower* her to *Satisfy* her senses of *Being* and *Belonging* that are enmeshed together in her role as a mother.

Summary

This chapter has explained the fundamental concepts of the *MOW* and how they work together in relation to *Health* and *Well Being*. Scenarios have demonstrated the application of the concepts through helpees' narratives. The main principles of the *MOW* will be expanded in the next chapter where *MOW*-based interventions are introduced.

References

Allen, K.-A. (2020). *The psychology of belonging.* Abingdon: Routledge.

Ashbach, C., & Schermer, V. L. (2005). *Object relations, the self and the group.* Abingdon: Routledge.

Cutchin, M. P., Aldrich, R. M., Bailliard, A. L., & Coppola, S. (2008). Action theories for occupational science: The contributions of Dewey and Bourdieu. *Journal of Occupational Science,* *15*(3), 157–165.

Del Fabro Smith, L., Suto, M., Chalmers, A., & Backman, C. L. (2011). Belief in doing and knowledge in being mothers with arthritis. *OTJR: Occupation, Participation and Health, 31*(1), 40–48.

Hasselkus, B. R. (2011). *The meaning of everyday occupation.* NJ: Slack Incorporated.

Hitch, D., Pépin, G., & Stagnitti, K. (2014). In the footsteps of Wilcock, part one: The evolution of doing, being, becoming, and belonging. *Occupational Therapy in Health Care, 28*(3), 231–246.

Ikiugu, M. N., & Pollard, N. (2015). *Meaningful living through occupation: Occupation-based intervention strategies for occupational therapists and scientists.* Whiting & Birch.

James, P., Nadarajah, Y., Haive, K., & Stead, V. C. (2012). *Sustainable communities, sustainable development: Other paths for Papua New Guinea.* University of Hawaii Press.

Jensen, S. Q. (2011). Othering, identity formation and agency. *Qualitative Studies, 2*(2), 63–78.

Lyons, M., Orozovic, N., Davis, J., & Newman, J. (2002). Doing-being-becoming: Occupational experiences of persons with life-threatening illnesses. *The American Journal of Occupational Therapy, 56*(3), 285–295.

Rogers, C. R. (1951). *Client-centered therapy: Its current practice, implications, and theory.* Boston, MA: Houghton Mifflin.

Van Huet, H. (2011). *Living and doing with chronic pain: Clients' and occupational therapists' perspectives.* Faculty of Health Sciences, The University of Sydney, Sydney.

Vansteenkiste, M., Ryan, R. M., & Soenens, B. (2020). *Basic psychological need theory: Advancements, critical themes, and future directions* (Vol. 44, pp. 1–31). Springer.

Yazdani, F., Nazi, S., Kavousipor, S., Karamali Esmaili, S., Rezaee, M., & Rassafiani, M. (2021). Does covid-19 pandemic tell us something about time and space to meet our being, belonging and becoming needs? *Scandinavian Journal of Occupational Therapy,* 1–10.

Further Reading

Bejerholm, U. (2010). Occupational balance in people with schizophrenia. *Occupational Therapy in Mental Health, 26*(1), 1–17. https://doi.org/10.1080/01642120802642197

Bonsaksen, T., Opseth, T. M., Myraunet, I., Hussain, R. A., Thørrisen, M. M., Ellingham, B., & Yazdani, F. (2016). *Hva gjør du i livet ditt?* [What do you do in your life?]. Unpublished manuscript, Department of Occupational Therapy, Prosthetics and Orthotics, Oslo and Akershus University College of Applied Sciences, Oslo, Norway.

Christiansen, C. H., & Matuska, K. M. (2006). Lifestyle balance: A review of concepts and research. *Journal of Occupational Science, 13*(1), 49–61.

Deci, E. L., & Ryan, R. M. (2009). Self-determination theory: A consideration of human motivational universals. In: P. J. Corr, & G. Matthews, (Eds.), *The Cambridge handbook of personality psychology* (pp. 234–240). Cambridge: Cambridge University Press.

Duan, C., Hill, C. E., Jiang, G., Li, D., Li, Y., Zhang, S., Yan, Y., Yu, L., & Lu, T. (2022). Meaning in life: Perspectives of experienced Chinese psychotherapists. *Psychotherapy, 59*(1), 26.

Edgelow, M., & Krupa, T. (2011). Randomized controlled pilot study of an occupational time-use intervention for people with serious mental illness. *American Journal of Occupational Therapy, 65*(3), 267–276.

Hammell, K. W. (2014). Belonging, occupation, and human well-being: an exploration. *Canadian Journal of Occupational Therapy, 81*(1), 39–50.

Harb, A., Yazdani, F., Rassafiani, M., Yazdani, N., & Nobakht, L. (2016). *Occupational therapists' perception of occupational balance and experience of its application in practice.* Manuscript submitted for publication.

Kielhofner, G. (2008). Dimensions of doing. In G. Kielhofner (Ed.), *Model of human occupation: Theory and application.* Baltimore, MD: Lippincott, Williams and Wilkins.

Klinger, L. (2005). Occupational adaptation: Perspectives of people with traumatic brain injury. *Journal of Occupational Science, 12*(1), 9–16.

León, J., & Nunez, J. L. (2013). Causal ordering of the basic psychological needs and well-being. *Social Indicators Research, 114*(2), 243–253.

Sheldon, K. M., & Niemiec, C. P. (2006). It's not just the amount that counts: Balanced need satisfaction also affects well-being. *Journal of Personality and Social Psychology, 91*(2), 331–341.

Stelter, R. (2022). Meaning as a topic in coaching. In: I. S. Greif, H. Möller, W. Scholl, J. Passmore, & F. Müller (Eds), *International Handbook of Evidence-Based Coaching* (pp. 553–564). Cham: Springer.

Wagman, P., Håkansson, C., & Björklund, A. (2012). Occupational balance as used in occupational therapy: A concept analysis. *Scandinavian Journal of Occupational Therapy, 19*(4), 322–327.

Wagman, P., Lindmark, U., Rolander, B., Wåhlin, C., & Håkansson, C. (2016). Occupational balance in health professionals in Sweden. *Scandinavian Journal of Occupational Therapy.* https://doi.org/10.1080/00016357.2016.1203023.

Westhorp, P. (2015). Exploring balance as a concept in occupational science. *Journal of Occupational Science, 10*(2), 99–106.

Wilcock, A. (1993). A theory of human need for occupation. *Occupational Science, 1*(1), 17–24.

Wilcock, A. (1998). International perspective: Reflections on doing, being and becoming. *Canadian Journal of Occupational Therapy, 65*(5), 248–256.

Wilcock, A. (2006). *An occupational perspective of health* (2nd ed.). Thorofare, NJ: SLACK Incorporated.

Wubbolding, R. E. (2013). *Reality therapy for the 21st century.* Abingdon: Routledge.

Yazdani, F. (2016b). *The occupational wholeness questionnaire.* Unpublished manuscript, Faculty of Health and Life Sciences, Oxford Brookes University, Oxford.

Yazdani, F., Roberts, D., Yazdani, N., & Rassafiani, M. (2016). Occupational balance: A study of the sociocultural perspective of Iranian occupational therapists. *Canadian Journal of Occupational Therapy* 26755045. https://doi.org/10.1177/0008417415577973

3 Understanding people and their narratives

Farzaneh Yazdani and Niayesh Fekri

Box 3.1 Chapter aims

This chapter will cover the:

- Significance of a helper's knowledge, skills and experience in understanding a helpee
- Strategies to facilitate a helper–helpee interaction
- Eligibility of helpees for the *MOW* intervention

The first step in planning an intervention is to understand the issues identified by helpees. Individuals or communities that are considered for a *MOW*-based intervention are believed to be those with problems around their *Satisfaction* with themselves and/or their life. There are some manifestations of *Dissatisfaction* in people's *Thinking, Feeling* and *Doings* that have to be focused on and explored further. People might be *Aware* or not of their *Thinking* and *Feeling* about themselves and their life. They also may not be *Aware* of how their *Feeling* of not *Being Content* might show in their *Doings*, the *Choices* they make and the way they respond to their situation. Manifestation of this lack of contentment could present itself more severely and might be associated with some diagnostic criteria for anxiety, depression or other types of psychiatric conditions. However, most of the time people who do not *Feel* content with their life and what they *Do/Not Do* have no mental *Health* diagnosis. The important point here is that a relative lack of *Satisfaction* and negative *Feelings* in people may be considered problematic when they have an impact on their *Motivation* for *Doing/Not Doing* things. Some levels of *Dissatisfaction* could be linked to growth and development and can be considered as *Motives* for further actions in life. A sense of *Occupational Wholeness (OW)* is achieved through moving towards *Doings* that help with *Life Satisfaction* and Self-Fulfilment. The problem starts from the point when people *Feel* uncomfortable with their life and themselves and confused about how to bring about *Change*. Some people might *Think* there is no possibility of *Change* (victim concept), others may *Think* it is not worth *Thinking* about it and so are not *Motivated* to take any action towards *Change*. Some people cannot differentiate the *Choices* they make based on their own *Capacities* on the one hand and the *Opportunities* and *Demands* of their *Context* on the other hand. *Context* consists of influential elements that contribute to how people *Think* and *Feel* about themselves and their life. *Context* has a huge impact on

DOI: 10.4324/9781003034759-3

the way people *Do/Not Do*. A deep exploration and understanding of the problem from *Individual* and *Contextual* perspectives is essential for identifying a problem in a person's sense of *OW*. There is also a necessity to learn whether there is *Congruence* or lack of it, between what a person might *Do/Not Do* in relation to their *Being, Belonging* and *Becoming* with what is *Significant* and *Meaningful* to them.

Equally important, helpees may *Feel Dissatisfied*, confused or distressed about either one or two and sometimes all components of *OW* regarding their sense of *Being, Belonging, Becoming* and *Doings*. They may express concern about the relationship between these components or the link between what they *Do/Not Do* and the association with their sense of *Being, Belonging* and *Becoming*. The helper should bear in mind that identifying these issues is based on their evaluation of the helpee's situation. Labelling the problem as such therefore is what a *MOW*-based helper does. Using the terminology of the *MOW*, the helper makes hypotheses to identify the problems.

The way for helpers to understand a helpee's problem is through an efficient use of *'Self'* by applying effective listening, responding and observing skills along with analysing people's narratives about their lives. The rest of this chapter presents the process through which helpers can identify a helpee's problem. To address this process, the following important matters are explained:

- Significance of helper knowledge, experience and skills
- Narrative reasoning as the most significant helping process
- Focus on interaction between helper and helpee
- Interaction centre intervention
- Identifying the signs that a person might have issues around *Satisfaction* with themself and their life
- A helper–helpee conversation and analysis

Significance of the helper

People may be relatively *Unaware* of their own state of *Being, Belonging, Becoming* and link these to what they *Do/Not Do*. This hiatus underpins the rationale for a third person's presence and helps to facilitate *Awareness*. The helper in the *MOW* has a significant role in establishing and developing a kind of relationship that supports a helpee's realizations of different aspects of their *OW*. *According to the MOW*, alertness about the link between *Doings* and each component of the sense of *OW* is believed to be key to the final perceived state of *OW*. Therefore, the helper's role in facilitating, encouraging and promoting the helpee's development of *Self-Awareness* in relation to their sense of *Wholeness* is crucial.

To implement this role, a helper is required to have certain characteristics, knowledge and skills to ensure the success of the *MOW* process:

- Awareness about their own interpersonal characteristics
- Knowledge and experience of people
- Knowledge and experience of efficient communication and professional helping relationships
- Skills in building and maintaining a professional helping relationship
- Knowledge, experience and skills in reflection
- Skills in helping professional reasoning.

Interpersonal characteristics

In general, helpers' *Awareness* about their own characteristics, assets and challenges in communication will help in any kind of helper-helpee relationship. Helpers are present in a professional capacity in the *Context* of an intervention. Their presence and behaviour, verbal and non-verbal, communicate messages to the helpee. Helpers have an impact on the way helpees present themselves to them and the way the interaction between the helper and helpee takes shape. Helpers' *Awareness* about their own interpersonal characteristics and potential responses that their behaviour provokes, encourages, facilitates or inhibits may be used intentionally. Apart from being a professional, helpers develop their own style that sometimes comes automatically to them in a helper-helpee relationship. Helpers should be alert and able to monitor their personal characteristics allied to their role as a professional helper. The personal characteristics of a helper can thus be employed within a professional role and boundaries as long as the helper is aware of them and when and where to present them and how they may guide helpee's responses. The *Intentional Relationship Model* (Taylor, 2020) is a unique source for demonstrating the details of helpers or in the terminology of the book therapists' therapy mode/style. Taylor's book is strongly recommended for helpers to enhance their knowledge and skills to aid them in a helper-helpee relationship.

Knowledge and experience of people

Helpers are required to develop knowledge in understanding people's characteristics and in particular their interpersonal characteristics that have a great impact on the way helpees communicate the story of their life. Knowledge of people is enriched by experience which can facilitate the development of skills required in a helper-helpee relationship.

Individuals' interpersonal characteristics are significantly related to several contributing factors that are almost impossible to determine fully for each helpee. However, the important point to consider is the diversity of both an individual's interpersonal characteristics and their expression of those characteristics. It seems impossible to understand all interpersonal characteristics given the breadth of variation based on age, gender, personality and culture. However, in order to establish and maintain an efficient helping professional relationship, helpers should value broad knowledge and experience of different people. Acknowledging the fact that people are unique in the way they are and how they experience the world is essential for becoming a culturally responsive helper. Through this, doors are opened to helpers who look forward to getting to know people and learning about them. Scenarios 3.1 and 3.2 describe situations that illustrate sensitivity of cultural use of language in communicating with others. The scenarios in this chapter are based on real stories with pseudonyms.

Scenario 3.1

Jessica, an MSc nursing student from Hong Kong, shared her story about a misunderstanding that had happened in the hospital where she did her practice. A hospitalized American tourist became critically ill and doctors suspected cancer. Blood tests were conducted for verification, but due to technical difficulties with the hospital equipment, the results were unavailable. Jessica went to the patient's room and began to explain by saying, "I am extremely sorry to give terrible news..."–. Before she could finish her sentence, Jessica realized that the now upset patient had understood her explanation to be in relation to the test results, telling them that they had cancer. Jessica said that by the time she had realized what had happened and tried to clarify the situation, the patient had become too distressed to listen. On reflection, Jessica *Thought* her use of the word 'terrible' had caused the misunderstanding, and that her intention to be extra polite and empathic may have been lost in translation. The patient was angry with Jessica and had told her that it was not 'terrible' news that the equipment was not working, and she should have just said there was a delay. Reflecting on the issue later, Jessica *Thought* that it was not only the word 'terrible' that had been an issue, but that perhaps because the event had happened in Hong Kong her intention and attitude were more open to being understood differently. While such instances are inevitable, Jessica said that it was a learning experience which encouraged her to *Think* more carefully about patients' characteristics and to predict potential issues that might interfere with effective communication, especially in sensitive situations.

Strategies to improve helpers' practice when working with diverse groups of people and their variety of interpersonal characteristics, especially with regard to relationships and communication, involve recognizing that each helpee has their own culture. Helpee's culture is identifiable by the way that they live their life and that helpers should be sensitive and responsive to the unique cultures of those helpees with whom they work.

One of the fundamental elements of effective communication with people from different social, educational and cultural backgrounds to one's own is to acknowledge that there is a higher risk of miscommunication and misinterpretation. It is crucial that the helper values the significance of effective communication as it is the essence of a *MOW*-based intervention. Furthermore, eagerness to learn more about the helper's own '*Self*' and culture as well as that of others is a crucial factor in succeeding in effective communication. It is necessary that the helper has a genuine eagerness/keenness to reflect on their own views, perspectives and likely prejudices. Through recognition of their own biases, the helper is able to pick up on difficulties or challenges in communication with potential helpees. In this way, they can identify likely obstacles that are rooted in their own issues instead of only focusing on the helpee's issues. This is the way to build relationships with helpees most effectively. Showing interest in the helpee's *Values* and lifestyle aid establishing a dialogue about their perspectives and allow for a more flexible approach where the helpee is also A*ware* of possible misunderstandings. Helpers should explain the rationale behind their eagerness in learning about helpee's *Values* and clarify that the knowledge of helpee's lifestyle aids establishing a respectful helper-helpee relationship. A helper's keenness leads them to be more observant and more receptive to the intricacies involved in communication with the helpee. A keen helper shows enthusiasm in learning about others, asks questions for clarity of understanding and naturally becomes less judgemental. Scenario 3.2 is an example of helper's appropriate use of language in showing interest in learning about helpee with a positive impact.

Scenario 3.2

Akemi is a carer of a 40-year-old man called Lewis who requires support setting up the equipment for his dialysis management at home. During a conversation, Akemi is not sure how to refer to the patient's partner who is also a man. Akemi is not familiar with the use of politically gender appropriate language and how she should refer to Lewis's partner. Akemi politely explains to Lewis that while her understanding of the language used between people of the same gender orientation is not familiar to her, Akemi is really interested to learn more about it. Akemi has just realized Lewis's homosexuality at the session when Lewis referred to his partner as "my husband".

Scenario 3.3 demonstrates a lack of interest in the helper that leads to ineffective communication.

Scenario 3.3

Ahmad, a Persian Muslim man, aged 50, is going to attend a group activity to discuss complications in fulfilling his sense of *Belonging* and strategies to manage them. Ahmad shows some hesitation in explaining his situation at first and then indicates that he is not able to attend the Friday sessions around lunch time that is a Muslim group prayer time. While Ahmad is not considered as a man who practises his religion, the importance of the Friday prayer for him is about *Being Together* with other people who *Feel Connected* to. The helper does not show interest in understanding the significance of the Friday group prayer for Ahmad and does not show any interest in knowing about it either. Ahmad was not encouraged to discuss the significance of Friday group prayer further. Ahmad *Feels* excluded from the group activity and finds it insensitive of the helper to not try and understand and help with the issue.

Drawing a comparison between Scenarios 3.2 and 3.3 should help acknowledging the importance of kinship and interest in helpers in learning about the helpee's world.

Akemi's example not only shows her eagerness but also her openness as a helper about her lack of knowledge regarding the use of gender-appropriate language. To present openness, helpers should facilitate a situation that allows expression of different *Values* and ideas respectfully and with no threat. A culturally responsive helper in Scenario 3.3 would pick up on Ahmad's indecisiveness in taking a decision and talking about the Friday's prayer time and its clash with the group activity that the helper was suggesting. The helper could show eagerness in learning about the *Meaning* of Friday's prayer for Ahmad and *Feel* confident and comfortable to discuss the issue with the helpee. One further positive step in Scenario 3.3 would be if the helper responded to Ahmad's strong *Motive* for attending the lunch time group meeting, validating the importance of this challenge for Ahmad. To validate the sensitivity of the issue of decision making for Ahmad, a helper would look into options that could facilitate Ahmad's attendance at the group such as negotiating the time with other group members or looking for other groups that may benefit Ahmad.

Key to respecting and consequently taking the best action when encountering a situation that challenges helper-helpee interaction is the avoidance of an attitude of right and wrong about culture and diversity. *Meaning* checking is advised as a good strategy to show eagerness to learn about others and present a positive attitude towards cultural differences.

Understanding helpees' narratives

Professional helpers should aim to understand those people who receive their services. No matter whether the helpee is an individual or a community, they have their own way of communicating their *Thinking* and *Feeling*. People have some understanding of their own *Needs*, *Wants*, wishes, preferences, challenges, assets and weaknesses. However, the way people perceive these features may not always cover all aspects as their perceptions might be distorted or hidden from their *Awareness*. Therefore, a helper should use all their professional and personal qualities to bring about an effective listening and responding interaction with a helpee in order to come to an agreement about their understanding of the helpee's state of *OW* or any components of their overall sense of *OW*. The narratives a helpee unfolds in their interaction with a helper are based on what happens between the two of them. Professional helpers must be sensitive about time and space they share with their helpees. To achieve this, the helper's application of appropriate listening and responding techniques should facilitate fuller clarification of the helpee's state of *Being*, *Belonging* and *Becoming* and the *Context* of their *Doings*. Nina's situation (see Scenario 3.4) later in this chapter shows the application of some techniques that assisted the helper in leading the session towards a better realization of the helpee's *Thinking* and *Feeling* and the *Context* of her actions. In summary, the helper gathers information which, together with the collaboration of the helpee, shapes the narrative. Therefore, it is necessary to check the narrative to reflect on the role of the helper in digging out the helpee's state of *OW*, *Thinking*, *Feeling* and *Doings*.

Interaction-centred intervention in the MOW

The *MOW* emphasizes on the interaction between the helper and the helpee. What a helpee presents at their meeting with their helper determines the process and content of the intervention plan. The helper's role is significant in enhancing the quality of the interaction, and as a result, the content and process of the intervention.

The quality of interaction is strongly influenced by the helper's role in:

- Facilitating helpees to express their issues from their own perspective.
- Facilitating a *Reflective* process for the helpee.
- Guiding the helpee towards identifying the links between their *Thinking*, *Feeling* and *Doings*.

The helper establishes the intervention based on what happens during the interaction. Hence, a successful interactive meeting provides concise and in-depth information about the helpee's *Thinking*, *Feeling* and *Doings*. The level of *Self-Awareness* about the links between the helpee's *Thinking*, *Feeling* and *Doings* and the contribution of these elements to an overall sense of *OW* is what this model focuses on. Therefore, strategies to develop and maintain an effective helper-helpee relationship are essential to ensure the efficiency of their interaction.

Strategies to facilitate in-depth interaction

Understanding the helpee's narratives during the interaction requires the helper's knowledge and skills of building and maintaining an effective helper-helpee relationship. There are many resources about strategies for establishing a professional/therapeutic relationship which emphasize communication skills. A wealth of resources is available to provide a reliable knowledge base showing the skills required for establishing an effective therapeutic helper-helpee relationship.

Being attentive and observant of the helpee's verbal and non-verbal language

In different stages of implementing a *MOW*-based intervention, the helper communicates the aim and fundamental concepts of the model to the helper. The helpee's understanding of the intervention process is present in their verbal responses to the helper's questions, how they assert their *Needs* and *Thoughts* and how they seek help. Helpees have different *Capacities* in understanding their own *Needs* and expressing them.

Responding effectively to the helpee's communication

According to the *MOW,* helpees may have different levels of *Self-Awareness* in relation to their own *Being, Belonging and Becoming Needs* and the ways in which these are linked to their *Doings* and within their *Contexts*. Raising *Awareness* about these links is one of the main aims of the *MOW* intervention. An effective input from the helper should facilitate exploration and discovery in the helpee's understanding of their *Needs* for *Being, Belonging* and *Becoming,* how their *Doings* are linked to them and how *Contextual* factors contribute to the interaction between them. Based on the *MOW,* intervention strategies are divided into two types: (a) *Empowering* and (b) *Enabling* strategies. Accordingly, the helper's responses to the helpee's narrative comments should facilitate implementing both of these strategies. Taylor (2020) explains the responding skills required in a therapeutic relationship that is equally applicable to the skills that helpers must acquire in the context of the *MOW*.

Employing strategies to facilitate the progress of interaction between the helper and the helpee

To *Empower* helpees to *Feel* confident in exploring their own life situation, what they *Do/Not Do* and what their *Doings Mean* to them, requires employing empathic and encouraging strategies that facilitate a collaborative relationship between the helper and the helpee. Acknowledging helpees' concerns and issues, challenges and difficulties is the most common initial step towards an effective intervention. Showing warmth and enthusiasm in understanding the helpees' world, facilitating opinion giving and sharing *Feelings* and *Thoughts* by allocating time generously allow formation of an interaction that facilitates the process of *Change*. While helpers should respond to helpees' issues with empathy, they have to take action at the right moment when the helpee is ready to move to problem-solving and addressing their situation. The helper and helpee discuss the options openly to find solutions. The helper should be prepared to respond to potentially strong emotions that may arise due to the helpee encountering realities about their own *Doings* or *Unchangeable Contextual* factors. Frustration and disappointment, often the most usual *Feelings* that appear during the helper-helpee interaction, should be handled through empathizing and encouraging strategies. *Encouraging* strategies are mostly employed to emphasize the helpee's strengths and previous experiences of success in managing difficulties.

To create an *Enabling Context*, the helper may be required to remind the helpee of their *Opportunities* and rights to access what they *Need* for facilitating *Change* in their situation. The overall principle of helper-helpee interaction is based on collaboration. To *Empower* the helpee for this collaborative interaction, the helper is required to apply the following strategies: to empathize, to encourage and to educate and raise awareness.

Strategies to empathize

To demonstrate empathy, helpers should use their verbal and non-verbal language that conveys a message about the helper's effort to understand or at least cognitively imagine what the helpee is experiencing. While representing empathy has cultural ground differences, there are certain principles that apply across cultures. Showing respect to the helpee and being non-judgemental, listening attentively and responding with warmth are all principles of empathy. However, how these principles are manifested in the helper's behaviour and verbal and non-verbal communication must be *Thought* of with sensitivity. For instance while shaking hands with helpees at greetings might be necessary in one organizational or community culture as a means to demonstrate respect, it may not be necessary or appropriate in others. Apart from the concepts that have to be culturally interpreted in order to facilitate conveying an empathizing message to helpees, there are certain techniques that could be usefully employed to establish an empathic helper-helpee relationship.

Paraphrasing the content of what the helpee says through active listening and reflecting on body language and *Feeling* all convey helpers' attentiveness to their helpees. Summarizing what the helpee says and when necessary asking questions that help to clarify the message, or probe to deepen understanding of the situation, would help demonstrate the helper's eagerness to know the helpee and care about their issues. Validating helpees' issues and acknowledging their difficulties convey a message of empathizing to helpees. Dismissing helpees' expressions of ideas and *Feelings*, underestimating them, moving too quickly to the next step of the intervention and giving advice all indicate lack of understanding.

Strategies to encourage

Helpers have to employ encouraging strategies to *Empower* helpees to contribute to the intervention and take *Responsibility* in exploring within themselves and what they *Do/Not Do* to meet their *Needs* for *Being, Belonging* and *Becoming*. Understanding the *MOW* terminology and philosophy and being keen to continue with self-exploration requires *Motivation*. Helpees *Need* to be supported while going through this process. This is important for helpers to remember that encouraging strategies are not simply the use of rewarding language and reinforcing words. Reviewing previous experiences when a helpee has been able to manage their challenging situations, identifying personal *Capacities* and assets and indicating positive *Contextual* factors as *Enablers* and supporters are among encouraging strategies. Providing a safe *Context* that permits open expressions of opinion, *Thoughts* and *Feelings* without fear of judgement encourages helpees to *Feel* more *Empowered* to *Make Choices* and disclose their *Thoughts* and *Feelings* about their *Choices*. An effective helper-helpee interaction necessitates this level of openness to facilitate helpees to exercise courage in self-discovery.

Strategies to educate and raise awareness

Building a helper-helpee relationship based on *empathizing and encouraging* is essential in establishing a collaborative relationship. However, to move the intervention process forward, a *MOW*-based helper should educate the helpee about the overall philosophy of the *MOW*. This becomes possible when helpees are ready to commit themselves to learning more about this model. The *MOW* helper then uses educational strategies in communication and reminds the helpee that at times they are required to be the learner, ask questions and practice intervention strategies. While there should also be agreement and collaboration throughout this educational process, the helper still has to use empathizing strategies at times when the helpee finds the learning process challenging. The helper also has to use encouraging strategies to *Empower* the helpee towards managing their difficulties with learning and applying the *MOW*.

Who is suitable for a MOW-based intervention?

The simplest and most straightforward response to the question of who is suitable for a *MOW*-based intervention is that it is an individual who seeks help for their *Dissatisfaction* with themselves and their life. An individual's or group's sense of *Dissatisfaction* with themself and/or their life is associated with their sense of *OW*. While people may *Feel Dissatisfied* with their life, they may *Feel* that they are making progress in completing their sense of *OW*. This means that a sense of *Satisfaction* within an individual's *Self* and with their world could be achieved at different stages and in different aspects of life. The sense of *OW* evolves through a person's lifespan. While individuals are always moving towards a sense of *Wholeness,* the *Satisfaction* with one's *Self* and life can happen during the process. To simplify this concept, a person would be *Satisfied* with themselves and their life and *Feel* that they are on the path towards their *OW*.

There are a wide range of reasons as to why people may seek help. Examples of such individuals are those who may *Feel Unhappy* or *Think they are Dissatisfied*. Some common expressions of needing help are given in the list below.

Examples of helpees

- Individuals or groups with no specific medical diagnosis who are facing challenges in their day-to-day lives. They *Feel Unhappy* or *Think* their life is not *Satisfactory*.
- Individuals or groups with a medical diagnosis who are also facing challenges imposed on them associated with their *Health* status.

Identifying indicators of Dissatisfaction

- Explicit expressions of *Dissatisfaction* such as a helpee saying, "I'm not *Happy* with my life", "I'm fed up with my job", "I am not *Satisfied* with myself/my life". In these situations, people are *Aware* of their *Dissatisfaction and/or Unhappiness* and use direct language to express it.
- Implicit expressions of *Dissatisfaction* such as "I wish I had a more supportive family", "I would prefer to be alone rather than being in a poisonous work environment", "I wish I had more time to spend with my child". In these situations, people may not be fully *Aware* of their *Dissatisfaction*. Alternatively, they may not *Want* to acknowledge their *Dissatisfaction* either for themselves or in front of the helper.

Regarding implicit and explicit indicators of *Dissatisfaction,* the helper should use their skills in probing and seeking clarification to ensure that there is a mutual understanding of what the helpees' *Dissatisfaction* is pointed towards. Establishing this mutual understanding takes place during the interaction between the helper and the helpee. This process may be less challenging when the helpee explicitly expresses their *Dissatisfaction*. However, there are situations in which helpees express their *Dissatisfaction* with one thing, but the dialogue leads to the realization of their *Dissatisfaction* with another thing. In the case of implicit expressions of *Dissatisfaction*, the first step is to reach an agreement with the helpee about the message that is conveyed by their expression, so that the helper and the helpee agree that the helpee is expressing *Dissatisfaction/Unhappiness*. Once the points of *Dissatisfaction/ Unhappiness* are identified, the helper needs to deepen their understanding of the helpee's *Thinking* and *Feeling* about the source of their now explicit *Dissatisfaction/Unhappiness*. Most of the time, there are multiple points of *Dissatisfaction* which overlap. An effective interaction would lead the dialogue towards creating a map that shows the links amongst the helpee's *Thinking, Feeling* and *Doings*. Through this mapping, the helper and helpee can build an agreement regarding the sources of problems which can then be prioritized and dealt with in the *MOW* intervention plan. In the next chapter, strategies to identify the problems that require addressing will be discussed in detail.

The types of *Dissatisfactions* that are addressed using the *MOW* are those that fit within one or more of the following categories:

1   *Being*: when there are signs of an individual's *Dissatisfaction* with the time and energy they spend on their own self. For example, making an effort to self-care, enjoying life and their own *Health* and *Well Being*.
2   *Belonging*: when there are signs of an individual's *Dissatisfaction* with the connections and relationships within their *Contexts*. This includes people, living creatures, places, objects and concepts.
3   *Becoming*: when there are signs of an individual's *Dissatisfaction* with their development and future prospects.

Helper and helpee interaction

Analysis of a conversation with a helpee is used in Scenario 3.3 to demonstrate a helper's skills and strategies in establishing points of *Dissatisfaction*. The rationale for the suitability of the helpee's issues to be managed using the *MOW* is also raised. The conversation is based on a real situation with Nina's (pseudonym) consent to use it.

Scenario 3.4

Nina, a 60-year-old retired music teacher, has self-referred to the helper (here, counsellor) to talk about her experience with her long-term neurological condition. At first, she started talking about how she was a very active teacher in the school and had *Control* over her own life. She used to spend time tending to her elderly mother who lives alone. Nina had an active social life and was very involved in the choir at her church. The dialogue below is part of the first session which started with Nina talking about the background of her illness and its impact on her life.

HELPER: Okay, so in the beginning of our talk you were saying that you started sort of not going to some of your social activities like your choir and focussed on your work (Helper summarizes what has been previously said). So can you explain to me in which way work was more important compared to other activities (Helper asks for clarification of the *Meaning* that prioritising work has for the helpee.)

HELPEE: It's just how I've been brought up that you go to work. This is what you have to do and as a teacher, you know in a school where there were seven classes of children. So you know the atmosphere was the one that you turned up for work you know, teachers turned up with a streaming cold and they'd still be there and I used to say, "you should be home with that cold, I don't *Want* it". But basically you know you had to be really ill to not turn up, it was just part of the ethos. (Nina appears confident and proud of how she presents herself as a committed teacher.)

HELPER: So you are saying that prioritising work has been a *Value* instilled in you. So what did it *Mean* to you when you had to stop working full time? (The helper explores Nina's interpretation of the *Changes* to see if there is any sign of *Dissatisfaction* about this.)

HELPEE: It was very difficult for me at first to accept to work part time. And even more difficult when I was forced to have an early retirement due to the severity of my condition. (Nina breaks eye contact, her body language becomes more inward, her voice has a more defeated tone.)

HELPER: So you are saying that it wasn't an easy experience to be retired while you were not ready for it? (The helper shows her understanding of what the helpee has said.)

HELPEE: Work *Meant* a lot to me but I had to give it up. I try to continue singing in the choir at the church. Every Christmas I organize a village choir and we rehearse for six Sundays leading up to Christmas and just contribute to the carol service … It always requires *Plans* for rehearsals and scheduling at rehearsals. But my ups and downs *Means* that I can't be sure about what's going to happen in advance. I pushed myself at times when my condition was flaring up because I *Felt* I had to go even if it was ten minutes. Sometimes I could get away with it but other times I couldn't. (Nina shows her frustration through her facial expressions. Her efforts to be part of the choir's activities show their significance to her.)

HELPER: I'd like to understand whether you continue with the choir despite your low energy because you enjoy it? (Helper probes for further clarification.)

HELPEE: I *Think* it's been part of my life. (Referring to something being part of someone's life, in this case participating in choir activities indicates the significance of it therefore the helper may need to explore this further.)

HELPER: So, I can see that the choir has been part of who you are and what you do. It's about the link between who you are and what you do. Am I right? (The helper shares her understanding and interpretation of what the helpee has said and seeks clarification.)

HELPEE: Yes, I've done the musical things, I've got my viola out of the loft, it's been there about 30 years, and I've, so I've been trying to get myself going on it to play it, and a sort of local friend has just started having cello lessons so we [inaudible plane passing by] get together and play duets, no matter how bad they sound, but I'd like to do that but I just *Think* I don't got the energy to go and do it at the moment, and it's, and lots of other friends I'd like to meet up and it's just difficult when you say, "well I can only manage half an hour when it used to be kind of an hour and I *Feel* like it's dwindling. (Nina is talking about something that she liked to do and at the same time shows her *Dissatisfaction* with the fact that she has limitations and has had to discuss it with others. Her limitations are part of the challenge, the fact that they are increasing is the other part of the challenge. She also finds having to explain herself to others difficult. In particular, when the situation is not stable and ever *Changing*. Her lips tremble and she starts weeping, she obviously *Feels* sad.)

HELPER: It must be very difficult to go through all these pains and fatigue when you're not knowing what comes next in order to *Plan* and communicate it with others. (Helper validates the difficulty of the situation and shows their understanding.)

HELPEE: Yes, it is really demoralising and when your situation keeps *Changing* and you have to *Plan* and *Plan* again and every time explain to others why I could be there for two hours last time and while one hour this time is beyond my *Capacity*. I can do things. I still try to be active but this is not the image I had of myself in this stage of my life, as if I am not a reliable member of the community, family or friend. Because me being there has ups and downs. I used to always be there for my mother, be beside my husband in his choir performing together and look at me now. I spend very little time with my mum, I *Feel* like I disappointed my husband with the *Plans* and dreams we had for performing in church together. (Nina is not *Happy* with the level of her participation in activities she used to do with her loved ones. She shows *Dissatisfaction* about her sense of *Belonging,* the way she *Connects* and *Relates* to her loved ones, and the *Plans* she had for her participation in the church community during her retirement.)

HELPER: I can see that you have applied strategies to manage your engagement with the activities and people that matter to you. I can also hear that it is not *Satisfying* enough for you.

HELPEE: Yes

HELPER: What does it *Mean* to you, not being able to *Do* the things that you have been doing before and in your own way? (The helper tries to get into the helpee's *Thoughts* about what she said and expressed *Unhappiness* or *Dissatisfaction* about).

HELPEE: I can't take care of others. It made my husband *Happy* when we used to work together but I can't do that anymore. I try a lot. I *Feel* useless. That's how I had learnt to be useful to others, by being there for them. I push myself but then my symptoms get worse. (It seems that Nina's sense of *Wholeness* as a person who can be independent, active and take care of herself and others has been affected by her illness. Her future prospects have *Changed*. What she had imagined herself to *Be*, a caring daughter and a supportive partner has been restricted. The current situation of her *Health* and its constant fluctuation has left her with little to hope for implementing her *Plans*.)

HELPER: Nina, am I correct in thinking that you are not *Happy* with yourself and the way you can be there for others? (The helper checks their understanding.)

HELPEE: Yes, that's correct. This is how I have always seen myself. But I am ill, I have very limited ability now to do things to support my loved ones. I have to *Think* all the time about myself and how to spend my energy to manage my own life. (The helpee explains how her limitations have *Changed* the way she was doing things, the time she used to spend on attending other's *Needs*, and her *Dissatisfaction* with the shift of focus to be on herself. She finds it difficult to do things that are solely for meeting her own *Needs*.)

HELPER: And what does that *Mean* to you? (The helper explores the helpee's perception of her current situation, her judgement and appraisal. The way she interprets the situation has an impact on the way the person *Feels* about it. And the helper investigates this further.)

HELPEE: That I am not the nice Nina I was. (This response represents the centrality of the *Value* that the helpee gives to *Being* a *Selfless,* caring and supportive member of her family and community. The sense of *Belonging* is a very significant part of her

Satisfaction with herself and her life. Her *Becoming* was *Planned* around the level of perfection with which she could offer care and support. Nina had associated her *Being* with her work and then after her illness, particularly in retirement, her church activities. Through this she could *Satisfy* her *Need* for staying engaged with the activities she liked (music, choir and children) and supporting people who she cared for. However, she is *Unhappy* with the level of involvement she can now manage.)

HELPER: I can see that you perhaps *Feel Satisfied* with yourself when you can *Do* something for others; your husband, mum, and children in the church choir? (The helper gets closer to identifying what Nina is not *Happy* about and brings it to her attention more explicitly.)

HELPEE: Yes and without that life I can't *Feel Happy*. (The helper and helpee reach an agreement on what the *Unhappiness*/lack of *Satisfaction* is about.)

HELPER: How about yourself? Who does take care of you? (The helper probes the helpee to *Think* about the way she views attending her *Being*.)

HELPEE: I don't know, I never *Thought* about it, I never cared about me and that's why I *Feel* so distressed now because all I *Think* of is me, my *Health*, my limitations and managing them. (Nina begins to realize how little she has previously attended to her own *Being Needs* to the extent that this attention due to her illness makes her *Feel* guilty and uncomfortable.)

HELPER: Could I say that your *Being* has been very much associated with how you could be of help to others who matter to you? (The helper brings Nina's attention to the fact that her time and energy for *Doing* things has been geared towards her sense of *Belonging*.)

HELPEE: I *Feel* my life has always been about others and not me. I *Feel* guilty about spending that much time on myself... as if I shouldn't...as if my *Being* has *Meaning* only if I can *Do* something for others. (Nina shows some signs of *Awareness* about the source of her guilt and the reasons as to why she *Feels* uncomfortable that she has to attend to her own *Needs* more than she would like to.)

HELPER: I *Think* we can agree that your *Dissatisfaction* with your current situation is to do with the fact that you have to attend to your *Being Needs* more than before and move away from your intention to focus on your *Becoming* and *Belonging*. Your sense of *Wholeness* has been compromised, as taking care of your *Needs* only for the sake of your own *Health* and *Well Being* has not been part of how you envisioned yourself and the path you had intended to take.

This interaction between Nina and the helper demonstrates how the helper's skills in communication and applying the *MOW* strategies facilitated the helpee to disclose her *Feelings* and *Thoughts* with the helper. The helper used strategies to show their understanding and willingness to understand accurately by seeking further clarifications. The helper encouraged the helpee to review what the *Meaning* of her *Doings* were to her and how she evaluated and appraised them as positive or negative experiences. Throughout the interaction, the helper was in charge of helpee's progress with identifying what they were not *Happy* about. This process of identifying the points of *Dissatisfaction* and *Unhappiness* occurred through the helper's responses to the helpee's verbal and non-verbal behaviour.

Next section presents a narrative that a helper and helpee wrote together using the *MOW* intervention. Wa'd AbuZuray is one of the *MOW* scholars from Jordan (see Chapter 13) who has worked as a helper with Enas, a young woman refugee from Syria, as helpee. Here is the narrative they have created together. Enas has given her consent to use her name and story in this book.

Enas–Wa'd narrative

On any weekday morning, the typical scene in Enas's apartment starts with the alarm going off at 6:30 am Jordan time. This is her cue that she needs to ignore the uncomfortable room temperature caused by poor apartment insulation and rush to prepare her seven-year old daughter for school before she gets herself ready for work.

Enas is a 24-year-old Jordanian lady who was born and raised in Syria, to a Jordanian father and a Syrian mother. At the age of 14, and as the Syrian war broke, Enas's family decided to marry her off to a Syrian man, in a step towards what they thought would protect her from the horrors of the war at the time. That's when the political war lost its *Meaning* for Enas and a domestic one started. Enas was in a physically and emotionally abusive relationship for seven years, six of which were lived as a refugee in her country of origin, Jordan, away from her parents and siblings. After seven years of violence and a child born to witness her mother being abused, Enas decided to get a divorce.

In an interview with Enas which focused on her sense of *Belonging*, we explored the key concepts of *Belonging*:

> Enas explained that her *Belonging* to both countries she had lived in is a mere state of *Togetherness* with both their societies. While she shared time and space with the communities on both lands, she does not recall a *Feeling* of *Belonging* to either country or to either people, neither as an adolescent, nor as an adult. However, in spite of not *Feeling* entirely "at home" in Jordan, she appreciates the fact that it is a safe place to live in, considering its political stability. A sense of familiarity has also helped her manage her life in Jordan, being the place where she grew up in into an independent adult; an adult who took the decision to leave a broken relationship and start a new life for herself and her daughter.

Being the strong-willed lady with a big sense of *Motivation*, Enas used all available resources and found herself a blue-collar job, which later lead her to re-starting school at a distant learning basis (home-schooling). This arrangement allowed Enas to continue her school education from her home after working hours, while she *Happily* embraces her role as a mother to her seven-year old.

Enas accepted the lack of social interaction in her distant-learning schooling system, with the hope that this will lead her towards a university degree at a later stage, where she can form relationships with colleagues and make friends.

Enas's employers have grown to become her friends. And although she doesn't spend much time with them outside working hours, she *Feels* like she can depend on them and refer to them when in need of advice or help of any kind.

On more than one occasion, Enas expressed interest in resuming school in front of her employers. Accordingly, they *Supported* her in getting enrolled in the distance learning programme, which had lifted her relationship with them to a new level of *Connectedness,* as they had supported her in pursuing an occupation which she highly *Valued*.

While her journey thus far had not been easy, Enas used all available resources and opportunities and created new ones which were not readily available for her, in order to make it work for herself and her daughter. Enas says that when the war broke, she was

---

Box 3.2 Activities for learning and reflection

Activity 3.1

• Think about a situation when a friend or family member was talking to you about their *Dissatisfaction* with themself or their life. Write down the conversation as much as you can remember. Now try to see if there were any *Being, Belonging* and *Becoming* issues in what they were communicating with you?

• Do you think the *MOW* could help them? In which ways?

---

young and could not face the world on her own. However, she now has the *Motivation* and the vision to work towards a better future. She *Predicts* this future to be with a small group of close friends, a degree and a well-insulated place that she can proudly call "home".

Summary

The significance of helpers' knowledge, experience and skills has been discussed in this chapter. Examples were used to help with learning about what a helper ought to know and act on based on the *MOW*. Readers were also advised to use other resources in which strategies and techniques compatible with what a helper has to acquire based on the *MOW* were presented. An in-depth example of an interaction between a helper and a helpee was presented to illustrate some of the skills that are required for establishing a mutual understanding of a helpee's issues that have to be addressed through the *MOW*. Finally, a narrative written collaboratively by a helper and helpee is illustrated.

Reference

Taylor, R. R. (2020). *The intentional relationship: Occupational therapy and use of self.* Philadelphia: FA Davis.

Bibliography

Adames, H. Y., Chavez-Dueñas, N. Y., Sharma, S., & La Roche, M. J. (2018). Intersectionality in psychotherapy: The experiences of an AfroLatinx queer immigrant. *Psychotherapy, 55*(1), 73–79. https://doi.org/10.1037/pst0000152

Barden, N., & Williams, T. (2006). *Words and symbols: Language and communication in therapy.* McGraw-Hill International. Retrieved March 12, 2022, from https://public.ebookcentral.proquest.com/choice/publicfullrecord.aspx?p=316251.

Boyd, C., & Dare, J. (2014). *Communication skills for nurses.* New Jersey: Wiley Blackwell.

Cohn, E., Tickle-Degnen, L., & Gavett, E. (1998). Therapeutic communication. *The Clinical Supervisor, 17*(1), 49–67.

De Rezende, R. de C., de Oliveira, R. M. P., de Araújo, S. T. C., Guimarães, T. C. F., do Espírito Santo, F. H., & Porto, I. S. (2015). Body language in health care: a contribution to nursing communication. *Revista Brasileira De Enfermagem, 68*(3), 430–436. https://doi.org/10.1590/0034-7167.2015680316i

Haynal, V. (2022). The coaching relationship. In V. Haynall & R. Chioléro (Eds.), *Coaching physicians and healthcare professionals* (pp. 30–56). Abingdon: Routledge.

Herlihy, B., & Corey, G. (2014). *Boundary issues in counseling: Multiple roles and responsibilities* (Third). Alexandria: American Counseling Association.

Lecca, P. J., Quervalu, I., Nunes, J. V., & Gonzales, H. F. (2014). *Cultural competency in health, social & human services: directions for the 21st century* (Ser. Social psychology reference series). Oxford: Routledge, Taylor and Francis group.

Morrissey, J., & Callaghan, P. (2011). *Communication skills for mental health nurses.* New York: McGraw-Hill Education.

Samovar, L. A., Porter, R. E., McDaniel, E. R., & Roy, C. S. (Eds.). (2015). *Intercultural communication: A reader* (14th ed. and 40th anniversary). Boston, MA: Cengage Learning.

Shealy, C. N. (Ed.). (2015). *Making sense of beliefs and values: Theory, research, and practice.* New York: Springer Publishing Company.

4 Identifying Incongruence/Gap, Disharmony

Farzaneh Yazdani and Niayesh Fekri

Box 4.1 Chapter aims

This chapter will cover:

- The analysis process of a helpee's narrative through creating *Actual* and *Ideal Triangles* and the *Incongruence/Gap* between them
- Examples of situations for using a *MOW* intervention
- The significance of *Meaning-Making* in understanding a helpee

---

Once an initial assessment has been done to ascertain a helpee's suitability for the *MOW* approach, the second step is to educate the helpee on the basics of the *MOW* using simple language. This second step frames the collaboration between a helpee and helper on the basis of their mutual understanding of how the *MOW* is to be used throughout the intervention process. Whilst the helper may have begun identifying the issues by linking the concepts of the *3Bs* (*Being, Belonging* and *Becoming*) and *OW* (*Occupational Wholeness*), the actual introduction to the *MOW* takes place in the second step. According to the *MOW*, a person's *Self-Awareness* about the state of their *3Bs, OW* and the links these have with *Doings* is the key to initiating *Change*.

Therefore, enhancing a helpee's *Self-Awareness* is a key strategy and the first stepping-stone for building the rest of the intervention. The *MOW* emphasizes the use of language and its impact on conveying the links between different components of the model to strengthen a helpee's *Self-Awareness*. Explaining the *MOW* in an accessible way by the helper depends on the cognitive and emotional status of a helpee. Therefore, the helper's professional reasoning and skills in communicating the ideas of the *MOW* are fundamental in this step. An example of the use of straightforward language in communicating the principles of the *MOW* is presented in the scenarios used further on in this book. It is important to introduce not only the components and concepts of the *MOW* but also their interrelationships. In other words, how one component links to the others. The second aim of educating a helpee is to *Empower* them to collaborate in decision making throughout the process of the intervention. Through this learning process, helpees are also *Empowered* to apply the same *Thinking* process to other aspects of their life after completing the intervention.

One of the concepts of the *MOW* is that individuals are constantly on the path towards achieving a sense of *OW*, and it is natural that *Changes* in their sense of the *3Bs*

DOI: 10.4324/9781003034759-4

Table 4.1 The MOW Concepts and Suggested Questions to Ask Helpees

The MOW concept	Questions to ask helpees
Doings/sense of Being	Do you *Think* you take care of yourself? What do you *Do* in your life to take care of yourself? What do you *Intentionally* avoid *Doing* for your own sake? Do you *Do* anything just for the sake of enjoying yourself? How much do you *Do* things that you like? Do you *Feel* you have *Control* over your life? Do you *Feel* you have *Autonomy* to *Make Choices*?
Occupational Wholeness	What do you *Think* about yourself/your life/the world? How do you *Feel* about your life/world? Do you *Feel Satisfied* with your life? What are your concerns about your life and the way it is going?
Doings/sense of Belonging	Who are the people/communities that you *Feel* you *Belong* to? Where is home to you? Is there any place that you *Feel* at home? Do you *Feel* there are ideologies/religions/*Values* you *Feel Connected* to? Do you *Feel* close/*Connected*/*Related* to people of a certain group? Are there any objects, places or anything that you *Feel* you have a special *Connection* to or *Relationship* with? What do you *Do* to make *Connections* with people/places/things you *Feel* part of/*Belong* to? Do you *Feel* lonely?
Doing/sense of Becoming	Who do you *Want* to *Be/Become* in the future? Where do you *Want* to see yourself in the future? What do you *Do* towards achieving what you *Want*/wish/dream of/hope for in future? What do you avoid *Doing* that would/could/might help you to get closer to your aims in the future? What do you *Do* to help yourself *Feel* more competent/able?
Actual Triangle	The *Actual Triangle* shows the links between what you *Do/Not Do* in order to meet your *Needs*. It also shows what you *Actually Do* to meet your *Needs* to take care of yourself, enjoy yourself, have time to yourself, *Plan* for your future and *Connect* to others.
Ideal Triangle	This *Triangle* shows your *Ideals*/dreams and wishes in relation to the way you take care of yourself, have *Control* over your life and the extent to which you *Feel* you have *Choices*. This *Triangle* is the *Ideal* way that you wish to *Connect* to other people/things and places. This *Triangle* shows the *Ideal* situation that you wish to move towards to meet your future *Plans*/achievements and who you *Want* to be in the future.
Reality/Tailored Triangle	This *Tailored Triangle* is based on the *Reality* of your *Capacities* and your *Contexts* to help you to take a step towards your *Ideal* situation.
Contextual Factors:	These *Factors* contribute to the way you manage your *Doings*
1 *Expecting*	1 Do you *Feel* there are *Expectations* of you to *Do/Not Do* certain things or in a certain way? What and whose are those *Expectations*?
2 *Demanding*	2 What do you *Think* of the home/family/community/workplace/school/friends, etc. *Demanding* what you to *DO/Not Do*? How do you *Feel* about them?
3 Restricting/Blocking	3 Do you find your *Context* of living/working *Restricting/Blocking* your *Doings*?
4 Encouraging	4 What do you *Feel/Think* about your *Context* in relation to your *Doings*? Do they *Encourage/Motivate* your *Doings*?
5 Facilitating	5 Do you find your *Context* Enable/promotes your *Doings*? Which facilities are available to you to ease your *Doings*? Do you use or could use these facilities?
6 Supporting	6 Do people literally *Support* you in your *Doings*? How do they present their *Support* to you? Do you find their *Support* effective?

occur throughout their life. Individuals, therefore, see themselves moving away from as well as towards their sense of *OW* repeatedly. Learning to apply the *Thinking* and *Planning* processes and what individuals *Do/Not Do* to *Satisfy* their *Needs* for meeting the *3Bs* is an essential skill integral to the *MOW*. Thus, while Step 1 is about identifying the point of *Dissatisfaction* and *Unhappiness* in a helpee's path towards a sense of *OW*, Step 2 is educating a helpee in order to establish a mutual platform for proceeding with the intervention plan. Table 4.1 shows examples of the questions that can be used to guide a helpee's *Thinking* using the *MOW* terminology.

Drawing different types of conceptual *Triangle* is a practical approach to facilitate a helpee's understanding of the *MOW* philosophy and *Practising Thinking* using the *MOW* concepts. First, by emphasizing what is *Actually* happening, the helper and helpee start drawing the *Actual Triangle*. Secondly, they draw the *Ideal Triangle* using the same template to identify the *Congruence* or lack of it (*Gap*) between the two.

It is essential to understand that *Incongruence/Gap* on its own is not a problem but that the problem emerges when other factors combine with the *Incongruence*. Below, the other factors that may be at play are presented with examples. All the scenarios in this chapter are based on real situation with pseudonyms.

Skewed Actual Triangle

Based on the *MOW*, neither of the *Actual* or *Ideal Triangles* needs to have even (equilateral) sides. Each side may be *Skewed* towards one of the *3Bs*. While a *Skewed Triangle* does not necessarily imply a problem, an exaggerated *Skew* over a long period of time has its own consequences for a helpee's *Health* and *Well Being*. Scenario 4.1 illustrates a congruent *Skew* between the *Actual* and Ideal *Triangles*.

Scenario 4.1

Mary, 17 years old, has been studying hard for her final exams at school. During the last eight months, she spent 10 hours a day, including most weekends, on her education and study-related commitments. She had little time for socializing. Mary postponed many activities and tasks which she likes to *Do* and which make her *Feel* good about herself. For example, getting a new haircut, going to nice restaurants with friends and ice skating which was her favourite pastime. Mary *Expects* her life schedule to be mostly the same for another year until she finishes high school. Her *Ideal Triangle* is in *Harmony* with her *Actual Triangle* for this period of time and at this stage of her life. She believes this is the way she can ensure getting the grades that will allow her to study her preferred course at university.

In this example, there seems to be *Congruence* between the *Actual Triangle* and *Ideal Triangle*. The consequence of a *Skewed Triangle* towards *Becoming* (over a relatively long period of time) may have a less negative impact on Mary's *Health* and *Well Being* due to her stage of life. From a psychosocial developmental perspective, planning and working towards future achievements are to be *Expected* at Mary's age. Furthermore, Mary is *Aware* that her temporary *Skew* towards *Becoming,* which is within a transitional period, is designed to push her through to the next stage of her life. She *Predicts* and hopes that by achieving what she has *Planned* for university, she will gain greater *Congruence* and *Harmony* in her *Actual* and *Ideal Triangles* in the future when she can spend more time and energy on *Doing* things towards both her *Belonging* and *Being* as well. Figure 4.1 represents Mary's *Actual* and *Ideal Triangles*.

Scenario 4.2 demonstrates another example of *Skewed Actual* and *Ideal Triangles* which, although in *Congruence*, may be more problematic than Scenario 4.1.

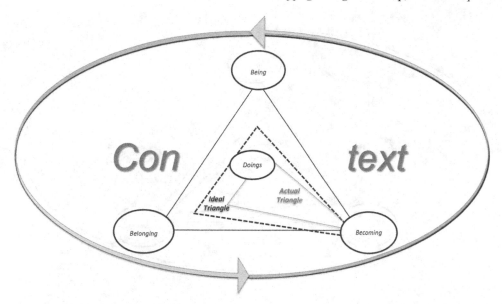

Figure 4.1 Mary's Actual and Ideal Triangles

Scenario 4.2

Ed is 58 years old and has had to take on a second job in order to pay off his mortgage due to the fact that his partner has had to stop working because of a *Health* condition. This *Change* took place a year ago and since then Ed has been working full time as a pastry chef in the day, whilst spending his evenings and weekends making food deliveries. Ed's *Actual Triangle* is *Skewed* towards *Becoming* in order to achieve his *Plan* to pay off his mortgage in the next 18 months. He has had little time to spend with his partner, which has put an end to their usual weekend outdoor activities together. He comes home tired and goes straight to sleep without having dinner. He has also been putting off his medical and dental check-ups due to *Being* busy or tired most of the time. This *Skewed Actual Triangle* has consequences for Ed's *Health* and *Well Being*. Ed, *Ideally*, would like to work less in order to spend more time with his partner. However, he cares little about not having time to *Do* his medical check-ups. Yet, overall, he still prefers to spend more time and energy on building a more comfortable future for himself and his partner. Moreover, he enjoys his current lifestyle as he *Feels* proud of making more money. As such, Ed finds the state of *his Skewed Actual Triangle Meaningful*. Ed considers giving up the time and energy to spend on himself a *Valued* sacrifice to achieve his goals. His *Subjective Well Being* indicates his *Satisfaction* with his lifestyle yet his *Health* is suffering. The issue here is that long working hours with no effective rest afterward and irregular eating habits have impacted his *Health*. Figure 4.2 shows Ed's *Actual* and *Ideal Triangles*.

In Scenarios 4.1 and 4.2, there are similarities between the *Skewed Actual Triangles* with different potential risks for *Health* and *Well Being* according to stage of life. Both Mary's and Ed's cases demonstrate positive *Subjective Well Being* that is represented also in the *Congruence* between their *Actual* and *Ideal Triangles*. While a *Skewed Actual Triangle* for Mary may have negative health consequences, these results may be characteristic of her stage of life. For Ed in a different stage of life, a long-term *Skewed Triangle* may cause more risk for his health.

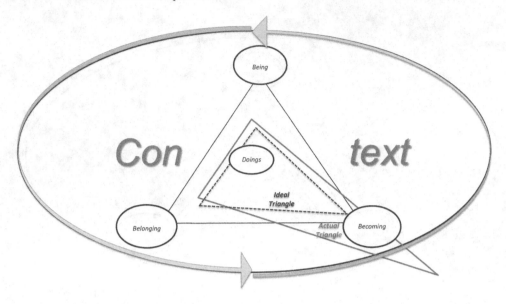

Figure 4.2 Ed's Actual and Ideal Triangles

Degree of Incongruence and layers of Meaning-Making

While excessive *Incongruence* between *Actual* and *Ideal Triangles* should be evaluated for its likely negative impact on *Health* and *Well Being*, *Incongruence* on its own is not necessarily a problem for *Health, Well Being* or a sense of *OW*. The significance of *Incongruence* is its degree as well as the person's *Meaning-Making* outcome. A small *Incongruence* may have a bigger impact on someone's *Health* and *Well Being* and sense of *OW* if a person has *Assigned* a negative *Meaning* to it. Alternatively, a larger degree of *Incongruence* can have less impact if the person has not *Assigned* a negative *Meaning* to it. It is important to note that following polar binaries of negative and positive *Meaning* is not useful as in many cases *the Meaning Assigned* to a situation has elements of both or neither. This suggests that there are times when a person may pay no significant or particular *Meaning* to an act or a situation. Most of the time, individuals evaluate a situation, *Make Meaning* and then *Attribute* a *Value* to their significance. This process has two dimensions that involve both cognition and emotion. For instance, a person may cognitively calculate the pros and cons of an action/situation and rationally reach the conclusion that the situation/action is overall a positive or negative experience. Although the cognitive interpretation of an action/situation has an impact on how an individual *Feels*, it does not necessarily ensure a positive emotion after a positive cognitive evaluation of an action/situation. The other point of consideration is that it is not always a positive *Assignment* of *Meaning* that leads to *Motivation* for action and a sense of *Meaningfulness*. This explanation emphasizes the role of narrative analysis in identifying the problem on which the *MOW* is based. Helpers are required to deepen their understanding of the degree of *Congruence*, its *Meaning* and impact on *Motivating* a helpee's *Doings*. The following two examples are used to demonstrate the above explanation of significance of *Assigning Meaning* in the way *Incongruence* between the *Actual* and *Ideal Triangles* may impact helpees' *Health* and *Well Being*.

1 Small degree of Incongruence

In Mary's scenario, her sense of *OW* seems to be based on what she was actually *Doing* which accorded with what she believed should be *Done*. Her *Ideal Triangle* was based on her *Expectations* which, for a young person who is planning for her future, were in line with the norms of her society. It is not strange that Mary based her *Doings* around an *Idealized* young person's lifestyle associated with the society she lives in. It is often hard to distinguish between societal and individual *Values* and related *Expectations* and *Demands*. However, in some scenarios, exploring this matter further is the key element in identifying a helpee's sense of *Satisfaction, Happiness* and overall *OW*. In Mary's scenario, she has internalized the *Values* of her society which she doesn't seem to be against. Therefore, it appears that there is *Harmony* between Mary's personal *Values* and what she deems to be her society's *Values*. Accordingly, the *Incongruence* between Mary's *Actual* and *Ideal Triangles* is small. Through her positive *Meaning-Making*, Mary justifies and *Predicts* her *Skewed Triangles* as *Enabling* her to achieve her *Doings* in the way she deems it should be *Done*.

2 Large degree of Incongruence/Gap

There are two dimensions to the analysis of a large degree of *Incongruence/Gap*. One is about the size of the *Incongruence/Gap* itself and the other is the *Meaning Assigned* to it. Generally, regardless of the *Meaning* that people *Make* and *Assign* to the *Incongruence/Gap*, there are consequences for their *Health* and *Well Being* which Scenario 4.2 demonstrates.

Scenario 4.3 is another demonstration of *Incongruence* in Evan's *Actual* and *Ideal Triangles* and the *Meaning* Evan has *Assigned* to that.

Scenario 4.3

Evan, 32 years old, is homeless. His *Actual Triangle* represents very little *Doings* in relation to self-care. He spends his time walking up and down the streets, his income is dependent on loose change from passers-by. He has made friends with a few of the other homeless people in the area, and they rely on each other's support. His *Actual Triangle* is a small one (see Figure 4.3). On several occasions, Evan has expressed a positive *Value* for working, and he believes that having an income can help him to have regular shelter, food, and security. He has also expressed that he would like to have access to a shower and clean clothing. He envies people who are able to help others by giving money. He wishes that he could support other homeless people as well as himself. His *Ideal Triangle* shows a big desire to *Do* things that can help him and his friends meet the necessary basic criteria to find employment such as clean clothes, a home address and bank details. His *Ideal Triangle* is a large one that is not in any way *Congruent* with his *Actual Triangle*. The large *Incongruence* shows the likelihood of physical and mental consequences. Evan sees this *Gap* as the result of social injustice and the government's bad management of issues around mental *Health* as he lost his job and home due to long-term hospitalization after his first episode of psychosis. Although the helper can validate Evan's explanation of his situation, they need to check what this *Means* to Evan. Evan *Feels* helpless to *Change* his situation in order to fill in this *Gap*. Therefore, what is observed in this scenario is not only the large degree of *Incongruence* that jeopardizes Evan's physical and mental *Health*, but also that the *Meaning Assigned* to this *Incongruence* by Evan negatively impacts the situation. The helper may agree with Evan's point of view but, according to the *MOW*, there are other ways to think about the *Choices* that Evan can *Make* within his very limited opportunities, to be able to lead a *Satisfying* life in spite of his restrictions.

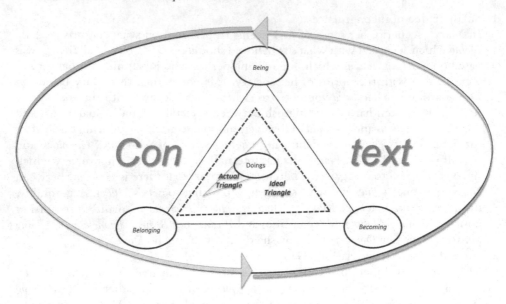

Figure 4.3 Evan's Actual and Ideal Triangles

The role and potential impact of Meaning-Making on Incongruence

Referring to Evan's scenario, the following questions can be raised:

At the deeper level of *Meaning-Making*, what does being a victim of social injustice and political failure *Mean* to Evan?

Could Evan *Assign* another *Meaning* to his situation and the large *Incongruence* that exists between his *Actual* and *Ideal Triangles*?

Evan has explicitly said that he *Feels* helpless to influence the government's policies and regulations that affect him. He *Feels* that he does not have many *Choices*. Yet, Evan's *Meaning-Making* is positive in respect of his everyday level *Choices*. For example, Evan *Assigns* a positive *Meaning* to being able to help other homeless people in his community. He *Feels* that his relatively *Healthier* physical state allows him to check in on others who may be worse off than him, he uses his time to offer support to younger homeless people. Consequently, even though the *Incongruence* between Evan's *Triangles* is very large, and its effect on his physical and mental *Health* is severe, he is able to soften its impact through the *Meaning* he *Makes* to the way he responds to adversity. Furthermore, Evan's religious beliefs feed into his *Meaning-Making* process. As such, in spite of *Being* a victim of social injustice by his own admission, he sees his situation as a test from God which provides him with an opportunity to help others.

Motivation

Evan's scenario shows how *Meaning-Making* is at the core of *Motivating* one's *Doings*. In the first level of Evan's analysis of the situation, where he sees himself as a helpless victim of external factors, he could as a consequence lose his *Motivation* for *Doing* anything towards fulfilling his *Needs* for *Being, Belonging and Becoming*. The significant role of the helper's skills in understanding the helpee's story is evident in Evan's scenario. Facilitating the helpee's telling of their own narrative has led to a deeper level of understanding of the *Meaning* Evan has given to his situation. It is apparent that the *Meaning* Evan has given to his role and responsibilities within the homeless community has been a source of *Motivation* for him. Therefore, while external obstacles inhibit Evan's *Doings*, his beliefs seem to be an internal source of *Motivation*.

Objectively identified problems versus perceived and subjective experience

The examples and scenarios presented in this chapter demonstrate how subjective experiences of one's *Doings* could be different from what is observed objectively from outside. At a surface level, drawing on the profile of one's *Doings* and how these *Doings* meet the *Needs* of the *3Bs* can be misleading. *Incongruence* between *Actual and Ideal Triangles* is not necessarily a problem. However, as the scenarios have illustrated, relying only on a helpee's perception of their own *Satisfaction/Dissatisfaction* does not offer evidence of good *Health* and *Well Being*. The helper's objective evaluation of *Incongruence* between the helpee's *Actual and Ideal Triangles* should be communicated clearly and effectively to the helpees. For instance, in Evan's scenario, his *Meaning-Making* to explain the large *Incongruence/Gap* between his *Triangles* is considered as an asset to help him to cope with his circumstances. However, a helper's evaluation of the situation signifies that such a large degree of *Incongruence/Gap*, in particular if it is over a long period of time, could lead to negative *Health* consequences. In this particular scenario, Evan's subjective experience of the situation is in agreement with the helper's objective analysis. Therefore, it is expected that Evan would collaborate with his helper to set plans to improve his situation. However, in Ed's case, Ed does not acknowledge the significance of the *Incongruence* between his *Triangles* and its potential impact on his *Health* and *Well Being*. This results in a disagreement between the helpee and the helper about how to develop the *MOW* intervention plan. There are situations, then, in which the helper may consider influencing the intervention plan based on a less collaborative approach. The following instances illustrate where such an approach may be applicable. First, when the helper's objective evaluation of the situation indicates life-threatening risks for the helpee. Second, when the helpee's *Choice-Making* results in jeopardizing the life and rights of the people around them. For instance, if the helpee's overall judgement is poor due to cognitive or mental *Health* impairments.

Harmony/lack of Harmony between Being, Belonging and Becoming

Another important point of consideration in analysis of the *Triangles* relates to the relationship between the *3Bs* and how a helpee's *Doings* towards any one of the *Bs* may jeopardize the other ones. The following examples may help in understanding this matter further.

Harmony between Being and Becoming and its lack with Belonging

Here, Scenario 4.4 shows how both *Harmony* and its lack may lead to issues in relation to a helpee's sense of *Self-Fulfilment* and *Satisfaction with life*.

Scenario 4.4

Zoya, 32 years old, is an artist who has spent a lot of her time producing a variety of paintings for different exhibitions. She has always been pulled by her own curiosity about nature. She has spent a significant amount of her time observing natural landscapes such as forests, rivers or mountains and their living creatures. Formerly, all Zoya's *Doings* were extremely focused towards how she considered herself to be a nature lover. She used to *Feel* more lively, energetic and creative when she was in nature. She envisioned that in/by her thirties she would be painting nature in a way that illustrated the less visible aspects of living creatures. Zoya focused excessively on achieving this aim (see Figure 4.4), she enjoyed taking *Control* of her activities and the time she spent on them by living in the woods, or seaside, or mountains. Throughout these years, after she had finished high school, she enjoyed leading a *Healthy* lifestyle by breathing fresh air, eating fresh food and *Doing* what she thought made her achieve her aims. While she *Felt* connected to nature, she had limited contact with friends and family. Initially, friends and family members would visit to spend time with her. However, gradually, the visits became more sparse as Zoya did not fully engage with her visitors as she was too preoccupied with her paintings. Recently, Zoya has been planning her new exhibition, and in the process of issuing invitations for a private viewing, she noticed that most of her friends and even her sister had turned down their invitation. She suddenly came to the realization that in all these years, she had not asked about them and that this had made her fall out of her previous social circles. Even though now Zoya is part of a circle of professional painters, she does not *Feel* that she *Belongs* to this group as she had never really made a *Connection* with people.

In the above scenario, Zoya's extreme focus on painting nature and her *Doings* to facilitate this, initially *Satisfied* her *Needs* for *Being* through fulfilling her desire to lead the life of her *Choice*. She autonomously structured her life around *Being* a nature lover:

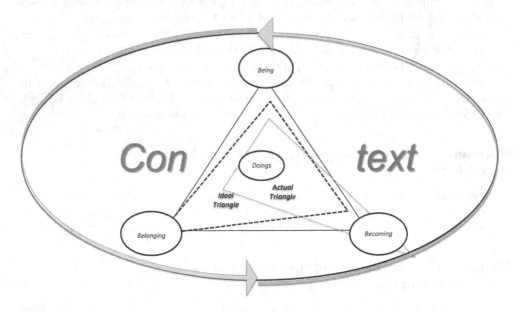

Figure 4.4 Zoya's Actual and Ideal Triangles

living in nature. She also extended her *Being* towards who she had *Wanted* to *Become* in her future: in *Being* an inquisitive painter of nature. Therefore, Zoya's *Doings* formed around who she thought she was and who she *Wanted* to *Become*. Her *Connection* to nature was an expansion of her *Being* that to some extent *Satisfied* her sense of *Connectedness* and *Belonging*. What she hadn't realized was the extent to which her *Doings* excluded the significant people in her life. Zoya had not considered that not sharing time and space and showing care for what others *Do, Think* and *Feel* had gradually separated her from her loved ones. Therefore, years before she had realized that she did not *Belong* to different groups of friends or even her family, they had already considered her as an outsider. Figure 4.4 illustrates Zoya's *Actual* and *Ideal Triangles*.

This scenario demonstrates how *Doings* that may *Satisfy* one or two of the *Bs* may threaten the other one(s).

Long term skews/exaggerated skew

Special attention needs to be given to the consequences of long-term and/or exaggerated *Skewed Triangles*. The theoretical assumption underpinning the sense of *OW* is that *Doings* should meet the *Needs* of the *3Bs*. Even though *Doings* may *Satisfy* each of the *3Bs*, this does not necessitate their being equal, although a fair amount of *Doings* should be specific to each one of them. It has been explained that a fair amount is unique to people's individual *Capacity* as well as their *Context, Opportunities* and *Demands*. However, to limit *Satisfying* one of the *Bs*, to the extent of eliminating it, has huge consequences for the *Health* and *Well Being* of a person or community. Scenario 4.5 illustrates Samita's story, an example of an *Actual Triangle* which has been exaggeratedly *Skewed* towards *Belonging* on a long-term basis.

Scenario 4.5

Samita is the mother of five children and the grandmother of nine. She was married at 16 in a society that strongly encouraged women to adopt a sacrificing role both as a wife and mother. She devoted all her time and energy to her children and husband. Her *Being* was very much defined around her role as a mother to the extent that she would easily ignore her *Health* and her *Needs*. She used to move from one bedroom to the other to check on her children at night, which indicates that she rarely had a good night's sleep. She would also make two to three kinds of meals daily to suit her children's and husband's taste and/or dietary requirements. She had no time for herself and she never considered her own *Needs* when budgeting for the family. Her *Being* had formed around the spiritual *Meaning* she had *Made* for her role as a woman. This *Meaning*, of course/ though, was aligned with the societal *Values* of the time and place which could *Satisfy* her *Needs* for *Belonging* to her own society. Her *Being* had extended towards *Belonging* to her family and society that praised her *Selflessness*. Samita's hope for her future was to see the joy and success of her children. Due to the structure of the society she lived in and what was then the norm of family life, she witnessed how the children and grandchildren gathered around grandparents and attended to their *Needs*. Therefore, Samita was not required to deliberately plan what she was *Expecting* from her future when she was older as this seemed to be an ongoing pattern in family life. At the moment, Samita is 78 years old and the society that she lives in has gone through dramatic *Change*. Unlike older times in which most members of the family would live relatively close by, four

---

Box 4.2 Activities for learning and reflection

The following activity aims to help you practise the language of the *MOW* which you would need to communicate with your helpees.

Activity 4.1

Consider Zoya's scenario (see Scenario 4.4):

- Write down how you would explain to Zoya what the *MOW* intervention is and how it can help her.
- Write down what you would say to explain her *Actual* situation in the *MOW* language.

---

of Samita's children live in other countries and the only one remaining in the same country as Samita lives in a city that is two hours away. From the age of 65, Samita has faced the new reality of rapidly *Changing* society. The economic and political status of the society she lived in had forced her children to migrate and work in time-intensive jobs. Samita's husband passed away. Her *Skewed Actual* or *Ideal Triangle* towards *Belonging* had to *Change*. She needed to attend to her own *Needs* as, unlike her parents' time when she and her siblings were tending to their *Needs*, none of her own children were able to do the same. Samita's *Being*, which was extremely linked to *Being* with and around her loved ones, is confounded by the fact that they are not there for sharing time and space with her. Samita had not practised seeing herself alone. The *Meaning* for her *Being*, which was the sharing of love and care within the close proximity of her family, had to *Change*. She had a lot of time on her own which she didn't know how to spend. She had not learned to plan anything that concerned only herself. Her *Becoming* was developed around her children's success and *Happiness* which they could not closely share with her due to the distance between their homes. The long-term and exaggerated *Skew* in Samita's *Triangle* towards *Belonging* has created a crisis for her.

Summary

Incongruence and the *Meaning-Making* associated with its impacts on people's sense of *Satisfaction* with their life/world and *Self-Fulfilment* were demonstrated through a range of diverse scenarios. *Skewed Triangles* were explained through examples to illustrate the formulation of the helpee's issues from the *MOW* perspective.

Further reading

Abdelhady, D., & Lutz, A. (2021). Perceptions of success among working-class children of immigrants in three cities. *Ethnicities, 146879682110221.* https://doi.org/10.1177/14687968211022114

Beike, D. R., Lampinen, J. M., & Behrend, D. A. (2004). *The self and memory* (Ser. Studies in self and identity series). Psychology Press. https://doi.org/10.4324/9780203337974

Boyd, J., & Zimbardo, P. (2010). *The time paradox: Using the new psychology of time to your advantage.* London: Rider.

Chandra, A., & Chandra, V. (Eds.). (2019). *The nation and its margins: Rethinking community.* New Castle Upon Tyne: Cambridge Scholars Publishing.

Jagieła, J. (2019). Psychopedagogy of self-fulfilment and autonomy: On the links between humanistic concepts and educational transactional analysis (part 4). *Edukacyjna Analiza Transakcyjna, 8,* 167–194. https://doi.org/10.16926/eat.2019.07.11

Lo, A., & Abbott, M. J. (2019). Self-concept certainty in adaptive and maladaptive perfectionists. *Journal of Experimental Psychopathology, 10*(2). https://doi.org/10.1177/2043808719843455

Martínez, N., Connelly, C. D., Pérez, A., & Calero, P. (2021). Self-care: A concept analysis. *International Journal of Nursing Sciences, 8*(4), 418–425.

McHugh, L., Stewart, I., & Almada, P. (2019). *A contextual behavioral guide to the self: Theory and practice.* Oakland, CA: New Harbinger.

5 Conceptualizing the Change that needs to be made

Farzaneh Yazdani and Niayesh Fekri

Box 5.1 Chapter aims

This chapter will cover:

• The use of *Actual* and *Ideal Triangles* as part of a helpee's narrative in identifying the areas that need to *Change*.

• How the rationale for the *Change* that is needed informs the aim of the *MOW*-based intervention.

Strategies for *Change* need to be identified by a helper in order to achieve the final aim of a *MOW*-based intervention designed to facilitate a helpee's sense of *OW*. Creating *Actual* and *Ideal Triangles* together with a helpee is considered the main means of involving helpees in all the steps of their intervention. Drawing the *Triangles* facilitates the establishment of a helper-helpee relationship and focuses the helpee's *Awareness* of their situation. Through drawing the *Triangles*, a helper creates a profile of the helpee's *OW* which, in turn, develops the helpee's understanding of how their *Actual Doings* inflect the *3Bs* of *Being, Belonging* and *Becoming*. The process ensures mutual understanding of the helpee's narrative. In Chapter 3, the dynamics of this interaction are explained through scenarios. The collaborative action of drawing a helpee's *Triangles* should lead to agreement on the *Changes* required to achieve the helpee's contentment with themself and their life. Realistically, there may be several areas that necessitate *Change*. Decisions about prioritizing the problems that require addressing, and areas that have to *Change* so as to manage those problems, depend on two main factors: the helpee's preferences and the helper's professional reasoning. Unlike the current emphasis of many professional guidelines and textbooks that underline the concept of client (helpee) centredness, the *MOW* emphasizes the centrality of helper-helpee interaction. The rationale behind this relates to the significance of the helper-helpee interaction through which the helpee develops a better understanding of themself. The helper, who also learns from this interaction, evaluates and re-evaluates mutual understanding of the helpee's problem. Therefore, the helpee's understanding of the problem and prioritization of their preferences for what to *Change* are based on a more in-depth understanding of their '*Self*' and their *Context*. The helper's background knowledge and experience are implemented through their professional skills in analysing the helpee's situation. The helper's

DOI: 10.4324/9781003034759-5

skills in communication and use of their professionalism in building the helper–helpee relationship guide the process of their interaction within which the helpee's *Self-Awareness* is raised. One of the significant skills of the helper in indicating the priorities of the helpee's problems is through developing links between different aspects of their *Doings* and their impact on the helpee's sense of the *3Bs*. The helper's knowledge of human science, including psychology and sociology, as well as the *Health* sciences that address body function and structure, guides the helper's analysis of the helpee's situation and, in turn, synthesizes a list of priorities for problems that need to be addressed. The following scenarios illustrate how the helper–helpee interaction draws on the helpee's strength which is rooted in their lived experience. Through the lens of the *MOW,* the helper's contribution to the interaction is based on their knowledge and skills to gauge the likelihood of causes and the factors which explain the problem. More specifically, the helper points to decide which aspect of *Change* is more significant and likely to be positively *Meaningful* for the helpee and whether the level of *Change* is *Satisfactory.* The helper also needs to consider two important questions. What are the *Changes* that should be made in *Actual Doings* that fit the person's opportunities and capacities? What are the *Changes* that might be made in the *Ideal Triangles* to bring it closer to reality? As a result of considering these questions, the helper and helpee develop a *Reality Triangle* which is a positive compromise or adjustment between the *Actual* and *Ideal Triangles.*

The art of analysis and interpretation

Interpretation of helpee's emotional and cognitive understanding of their *Actual* and *Ideal* situation is essential in conceptualizing what needs to *Change.* Each helpee has a way of looking at their problems through their own analysis. A helper should learn what the helpee's analysis is and how they explain their problem. How the problem is perceived by a helpee represents what their emotional and cognitive appraisal of the situation is and how, in turn, this matter has informed their responses to the situation. How the helpee emotionally and cognitively demonstrates their story is core to the helper's understanding of them. While helpers have their own analysis of the situation, the helpee's point of view is central to what the problem is and how the helper–helpee interaction informs the *MOW* intervention plan. The role of the interaction between the helpee and the helper is explained in Chapter 3. In this chapter, the helpee's emotional and cognitive presentation of their issues is discussed in more depth starting with Alexandra's case in Scenario 5.1. All scenarios in this chapter are based on real situations with pseudonyms.

Scenario 5.1

Alexandra, a 24-year-old student, works hard and is engaged in a lot of *Doings* to ensure high academic achievement. Her *Actual* and *Ideal Triangles* show *Incongruence* illustrating a large *Skew* towards her *Becoming.* Although Alexandra has indicated that she has achieved high marks in all her studies, she is still *Unhappy* about her *Becoming.* She has been neglecting her self-care and she doesn't spend any time with her family and friends. As a result, her *Actual Triangle* is severely *Skewed* towards her *Becoming.* In her analysis of her own situation, she does not find any problem with ignoring her needs for *Being* and *Belonging.* The *Change* in her situation that Alexandra identifies is to engage with strategies that will help her to invest in more *Doings* that will ensure further achievement and success. In the helpee–helper interaction, the helper tries to understand the *Meaning* of further achievements and success from Alexandra's perspective. In Alexandra's story, she mentions how her parents are considered successful and high achieving academics and how they had always hoped that Alexandra would follow in their footsteps. When probing further into Alexandra's *Feelings,* the helper realizes that what matters to Alexandra is not the achievement itself: it is actually the approval of her parents. Alexandra mentions how at times in their social circles, her parents insisted on bringing Alexandra's success to their friends' attention and how this has deeply influenced Alexandra's *Being.* Alexandra's internalization of her own worth is associated with accomplishment and her *Belonging* is dependent on her parents' approval of her *Doings.* Alexandra has grown up in a context of high *Expectations* which demanded of her the expenditure of much time and energy. The helper's interpretation of Alexandra's situation was that her *Doings* are guided by her huge *Need* for *Feeling* worthy. She *Wanted* her parents to feel proud of her. She hoped to *Connect* with her parents' high achieving circle of friends. The helper interpreted that Alexandra's *Doings* are to ensure she can be part of that group, in order to *Relate* to them, and to *Feel* like she *Belongs.* When the helper probed for the *Meaning* of success from Alexandra's perspective, Alexandra found difficulty in separating what success *Means* to her without reference to what it *Means* to her parents. Alexandra became very *Emotional* when talking about her parents' disappointment when she wasn't accepted by the premier university in their country to study medicine and had to enrol at a less prestigious university. She explained to the helper the pressure her parents were under in their social circle and how they did not *Want* to bring the topic up in their gatherings with them afterwards. The helper, therefore, needing to bring her own evaluation of the problem to Alexandra's attention, said that the problem with her *Triangles* was not about the *Gap* between her *Actual* and *Ideal Becoming* but about the lack of Alexandra's *Awareness* regarding the *Meaning* of her *Doings* in relation to her *Being* and *Belonging.* In other words, Alexandra had never considered that all the time and energy she spends on *Doings* to ensure her *Becoming* is actually to satisfy her sense of *Being* a competent individual approved by her parents. It was not in Alexandra's *Awareness* that she was yearning for her parents' approval and *Needs* for *Belonging.*

This scenario highlights the significance of the helper–helpee relationship through identifying what the problem is and what needs to *Change.* According to Alexandra's analysis of her own situation, moving towards who she had *Wanted* to *Be* in the future and who she had *Wanted* to *Become* had established the necessity of *Doing* more to achieve more. Whilst achievement did not have a particularly *Satisfying Meaning* to her, it was only in conversation with the helper that she realized she did not have a distinct sense of her own *Becoming.* While Alexandra had said her *Being* and *Belonging* were not points of concern for her, it was only in conversation with her helper that she realized the significance of her *Needs* for *Being* and *Belonging.* As a result of this interaction, Alexandra and her helper agreed to *Reflect* on Alexandra's *Doings* which informed the deep but explicit *Meaning* of *Doings* as a means for success. In summary, Alexandra's problem is her lack of *Awareness* about the influence of her *Needs* for *Belonging* and *Being* which revealed itself in her emotional responses. The *Meaning* Alexandra *Made* for her *Doings* and the *Values* she *Attributed* to them are the key problems that Alexandra's scenario presents. What is necessary to *Change,* therefore, is Alexandra's insight about the *Meaning* of her *3Bs* and the interactions among them in order to be able to draw an *Actual* and *Ideal Triangle* that is closer to the truth of her situation.

The starting points of Change

Once the helper has made a hypothesis locating the problematic areas, and a mutual understanding of the situation reached through discussion with the helpee, it is time to decide how to begin the process of *Change*. The where, when, how and who of *Change* are all key points of consideration. According to the *MOW,* the means of *Change* is through *Doings*; however, decisions about which *Doings* and how they may cause *Change* are other significant matters in the helping process. As all components are interrelated, any *Change* in one is expected to have an impact on others. For this reason, it is essential to identify what kind of *Change* is fundamental, practical and likely to happen within a helpee's *Capacity* over a considered period of time. To design such a *Change* in a helpee's *Doings,* their potential *Individual Capacities, Contextual Factors* and, in particular, their access to resources must be carefully examined, explored and planned.

Understanding a person's view of the world and themself

People generally *Plan* their life based on how they see themselves within their own world. An individual's understanding of themself is in different levels of proximity to their true *Self* while their *Plans* for living and how to pursue their *Plans* depend on this understanding. An individual's understanding of their *Capacities* (emotional, physical and cognitive) for *Doings* encourages them to initiate action. The individual's worldview and how they see themselves within their *Context* is another factor in the initiation of any action. For instance, in the case of Alexandra (Scenario 5.1), she sees *Value* in her achievements, and her self-worth (italics?) is based on her *Being* an achiever. Her worldview is that successful people are well respected and accepted by society and so she puts all of her energy into gaining that respect from significant people in her life. To Alexandra, the *Meaning* of life is to be seen as an accomplished person by others. In contrast, the next scenario (Scenario 5.2) shows how Masha's views of life and herself are completely different from Alexandra's.

Scenario 5.2

Masha is 15 years old. She believes that she has musical talent as she has been given positive feedback from her friends, family and, in particular, in school from her teachers. She has achieved several awards for her performance in school and in local music events. She likes playing music, and she believes that it is an important skill to have. The *Context* she lives in consists of several people who are *Supportive* of her; she has good resources and funds to *Facilitate* her further education in music. However, her worldview and how she views herself within that seem to be different. She appreciates music but she does not count on success in playing music as part of her existential *Values*. She believes that each individual should help oppressed and disadvantaged people. She sees the world as a place that gives people opportunities to work towards making it a better place to live, and she *Wants* to take action to *Do* that rather than trying to *Be* a successful musician. Masha's parents think that she is an emotional young woman who will regret her decision if she doesn't pursue music which provides her with a road for success, prosperity, and fame. However, Masha, at this stage of her life, sees herself as an empathetic individual who is able to put her time and energy into something that can address the *Needs* of people less privileged than herself.

In this scenario, Masha has all the elements of *Support* to sustain the *Doings* necessary to ensure her path towards *Being* a musician; however, this is not how she sees herself now. A strong contributing factor to Masha's decision about her *Doings* rests on how she *Values* being engaged in activities other than her music. Her understanding of what her music activities may bring to her and how they could build her future doesn't seem to *Satisfy* her wish of helping people in need and therefore does not contribute to her sense of *Becoming*.

The next scenario introduces how scoring a helpee's *Triangles* may help with *Reflecting* on *Changes* as the helper and helpee progress through a *MOW*-based intervention. In Scenario 5.4, a helper identified the suitability of Ayda, a helpee, for a *MOW*-based intervention. The helper and helpee draw *Actual* and *Ideal Triangles* which they jointly score. Scoring is part of the process to help quantify a helpee's sense of their *3Bs*. Through this process, *Changes* become more objective and noticeable. Scoring the *Triangles* is explained next.

How to score Actual and Ideal Triangles

The *Hypothetical, Actual, Ideal* and *Tailored (Reality) Triangles* were introduced in Chapter 2. Each *Triangle* has three apexes and three sides. The apexes, respectively, indicate *Being, Belonging* and *Becoming*.

Each Triangle has three sides: *Being-Belonging, Being-Becoming* and *Belonging-Becoming*. At the centre of each *Triangle* is *Doings*, a line can be drawn from each apex to *Doings* to show the relationship between each *B* and *Doings*.

In the scoring system, the *Doings* at the centre are scored zero. Helpees can score themselves as to how they *Think* their *Doings* meet their *Needs* for each one of the *Bs*. The score ranges between +10 at the apex of the *Hypothetical Triangle* to indicate the highest level of satisfaction with *Doings* related to each of the *Bs*. For instance, if a person thinks what they DO/Not Do fully *Satisfies* their sense of *Being*, then in their *Actual Triangle* they self-score it as +10 while −10 is used to indicate the lowest level of *Satisfaction*. The same scoring process applies to each of the *3Bs*. If a person *Thinks* their *Doings* make them take more distance from where and with whom they *Feel* a sense of *Belonging*, their score may range from −1 to −10 depending on how *Dissatisfied* they find their situation. The most extreme expression of *Dissatisfaction* would be if a person were to score all *3Bs* at the extreme end of the negative scale on their *Actual Triangle* but plot extreme positive scores on their *Ideal Triangle*.

Another example of extreme self-scoring is when both *Actual* and *Ideal Triangles* are on the negative side of the scale in each of the *3Bs*. In such a situation, a person's *Doings* show that their *Actual Doings* are not *Satisfying* them but that they have neither wish nor *Expectation* for *Change*.

Scenario 5.3 outlines/describes/presents a real situation that demonstrates an extreme situation in a helpee's *Actual* and *Ideal Triangles*. Pseudonyms have been used to protect anonymity.

Scenario 5.3

Simon is homeless and a rough sleeper, doesn't eat well and has no family around. He prefers to stay on the same street and doesn't like to go elsewhere in the city. He *Feels* a sense of togetherness with other people who live on the same street but doesn't talk to them and keeps himself to himself. He has five children and misses them but *Feels* they abandoned him following his discharge from a mental *Health* hospital. To meet his sense of *Belonging,* Simon's *Doings* are limited to staying on the same street where he feels safe and relatively secure. He doesn't identify anything that might help his future and has no *Expectation* of *Change,* either. He wishes to see his children, and this is the only reason which attracts a positive score in his *Ideal Triangle.* Simon would like to make a *Change* to his *Doings* to help him to see his children. He wishes to *Do* things that would help him to live in a shelter and sleep in a better bed. He likes to *Think* of a better life that would meet his basic *Needs* for more regular food, a clean bed and a warm place in winter. Figure 5.1 shows Simon's *Actual* and *Ideal Triangles* with his scores.

Simon's *Actual Triangle* scores:

Being: −4, Belonging: −8, Becoming: −10
Simon's *Ideal Triangle* scores:

Being: +3, Belonging: +3, Becoming: 0

Figure 5.1 shows an example of scoring the *Actual* and *Ideal Triangle* of a helpee with a high level of *Dissatisfaction* with *Doings* towards *3Bs* in the *Actual Triangle.* The *Ideal Triangle* is scored extremely low as well which indicates a low *Expectation* of *Change* in this helpee. Such extreme *Triangles* should be alarming for both helper and helpee, and it might be that the helpee needs referral to other services such as psychotherapy and social services.

Scenario 5.4 demonstrates the way Ayda and her helper agree on *Changes* and *Plan* for them.

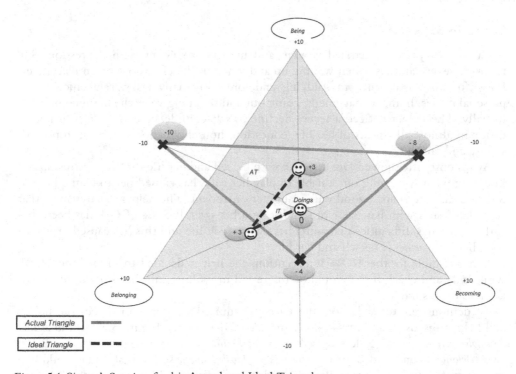

Figure 5.1 Simon's Scoring for his Actual and Ideal Triangles

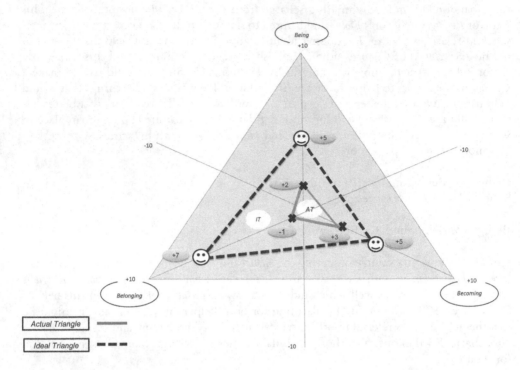

Figure 5.2 Ayda's Actual and Ideal Triangles

Scenario 5.4

Ayda is a 26-year-old married woman and university student with depression. She reported severe anxiety when waking up and when in the classroom or on placement. Forgetfulness, disturbance in studying and forgetting daily tasks, reluctance to do personal duties, home management, going out and shopping were the main complaints initially. The helper noticed a severe decline in self-confidence and *Feelings* of inadequacy in almost all aspects of her life (education, household chores, relationships with spouse and family).

Ayda constantly showed *Dissatisfaction* with herself and her life through distress in not knowing what was going on. Unable to play her roles has caused her to blame herself. She says that she is not a good wife, daughter or student. The helper's analysis was that Ayda has issues with her *Sense of the 3Bs,* and her overall *Sense of OW* has been disturbed. She has difficulties managing her day-to-day life and this has caused problems with her *Satisfaction* of herself and her life.

Being eligible for the *MOW* intervention, the helper decided to discuss the *MOW* with Ayda and check if she would be interested in looking into her situation through the lens of this model.

To demonstrate to Ayda how the *Changes* required are conceptualized, the helper and helpee discussed and drew *Actual* and *Ideal Triangles* (see Figure 5.2). In the *Actual Triangle*, Ayda gave the following scores to her *Doings* in relation to her *Needs* for *Being*: two, *Belonging*: one, and *Becoming*: three. Her *Ideal Triangle* shows that Ayda would like to achieve five in *Being*, five in *Becoming* and seven in *Belonging*. By drawing the *Triangles*,

Ayda came to see how far she is from her desired situation. She was asked to set goals for each of the areas. The helper and Ayda agreed on step-by-step *Changes* to her situation, indicating the contributing factors to the current situation as well as their roles in the necessary *Changes* to be made. Together with her helper, Ayda identified that the biggest obstacles to making *Changes* were her beliefs about herself in relation to *Meaning-Making and Attributing Values* to her own characteristics and *Doings*. For instance, Ayda *Attributes Value* to self-worth based on errorless performance in all her roles. In brief, it was agreed that the *MOW* intervention for Ayda needs to focus on *Facilitating Changes* in her attitude towards herself and the world, *Expectations* and *Meaning-Making* for her *Doings* as well as *Attributing Values* to her *Doings*. To achieve this, Ayda and her helper agreed to *Change* her *Doings* through different *Choice-Making* in day-to-day actions.

Summary

The significance of helper-helpee relationships in understanding a helpee's situation and identifying problems were presented in scenarios to help readers grasp how a *MOW*-based intervention is informed by the helper-helpee interaction and the way that *Actual* and *Ideal Triangles* facilitate this process. Drawing *Actual* and *Ideal Triangles* and scoring them was explained using one example.

Box 5.2 Activities for learning and reflection

To practise conceptualizing the *Changes* needed by a helpee, look at the following scenario and write an analysis of the situation. Show your reasoning as a helper to conceptualize what needs to *Change*.

Marivan is a 46-year-old worker who used to spend 10 hours a day on building construction sites. His income was satisfactory for his small family. Marivan was proud of himself for being able to manage his family life after moving from his village to the capital city. Recently he had a stroke and is not able to keep his balance and walk around easily. Marivan's employer has informed him that the company cannot pay him anymore as his sick leave has gone beyond six months. Marivan finds it difficult to believe that he has lost his physical *Capacity* for working at the company. He has no insurance to cover his living costs. He has lost respect for himself as he feels he is not useful to his family. He does not talk to his daughter and wife and avoids appearing in public. His mind is preoccupied with his losses and Marivan thinks he should go back to where he was in his life and denies that his situation has changed.

- What do you think are the *Incongruences* between Marivan's *Actual* and *Ideal Triangles*?

- What is your hypothesis to explain his difficulties and *Dissatisfaction* with himself and his life?

- How would you approach Marivan and interact with him about his situation?

Further Reading

Brandes, B., & Lai, Y. L. (2022). Addressing resistance to change through a micro interpersonal lens: An investigation into the coaching process. *Journal of Organizational Change Management, 35*(3), 666–681.

Haynal, V. (2022). The coaching relationship. In: Haynal, V., and Chioléro, R. (Eds) *Coaching physicians and healthcare professionals* (pp. 30–56). Abingdon: Routledge.

Mee, J., & Sumsion, T. (2001). Mental health clients confirm the motivating power of occupation. *British Journal of Occupational Therapy, 64*(3), 121–128.

Ryan, R. M., Lynch, M. F., Vansteenkiste, M., & Deci, E. L. (2011). Motivation and autonomy in counseling, psychotherapy, and behavior change: A look at theory and practice 1ψ7. *The Counseling Psychologist, 39*(2), 193–260.

Smith, M. L., Van Oosten, E. B., & Boyatzis, R. E. (2009). Coaching for sustained desired change. *Research in organizational change and development. 17,* 145–173.

6 Identifying the helpees' Readiness for Change (Change plan and implementation process)

Farzaneh Yazdani

Box 6.1 Chapter aims

This chapter will cover:

- The *MOW*-based intervention in three phases
- Evaluating the helpee's *Readiness* for a *MOW*-based intervention
- Aspects of a helpee's view of themself and the world
- Aspects of *Doings* that can be considered appropriate for *Change*

Helpees in a *MOW*-based intervention may be an individual or group of people. The *MOW* intervention plan differs depending on the individual's/community group's *Readiness* for initiating the process of *Change*. This chapter first explains how to evaluate the individual helpee's *Readiness* for *Change* in three phases: phase I—initial encounter, phase II—evaluating eligibility and *Readiness* and phase III—*Change* process. Then, the three phases are explained in relation to helpees as a community group.

Evaluating an individual helpee's Readiness for a MOW-based intervention

It is important to acknowledge the significance of the helper-helpee relationship in facilitating the entire journey from phases I to III.

- Phase I
  Phase I of the intervention is to hold the initial interview to indicate if the helpee's issues are suitable to be explored through the lens of the *MOW*. Self-referral is perhaps the most obvious sign of *Readiness*. However, individuals may identify that there is a problem they *Want* to address but refer themselves to the wrong services or with the wrong *Expectations*.
- Phase II
  Phase II starts with evaluating the helpee's *Awareness* about their *Actual* and *Ideal Triangles* through the filters of *Being, Belonging* and *Becoming (3Bs)* and investigating their *Satisfaction* and *Dissatisfaction* with *Self*/life and the world.

DOI: 10.4324/9781003034759-6

Table 6.1 The MOW Concepts in Lay Language

The MOW theoretical concept	The MOW concept in lay language
Occupational Wholeness	It's an evaluation of life situations when you are *Satisfied* with your life situation and *Feel* relatively good about it.
Doings	Your actions, what you *Intentionally Do* or *Not Do*.
Being	The way you see yourself, what you like and what makes you genuinely *Happy,* gives you a sense of joy, makes you *Feel* you have *Control* over your own life, you can *Choose*.
Belonging	Who you like to be with, spend time with, share space with. Place you enjoy or *Value* to be, where you like to visit, *Feel* at home, ideas you *Think* define your *Values*, people/places, ideas you *Feel* part of.
Becoming	Your future *Plan,* what you hope for, where you *Want* to be in future, who you would like to *Become*.
Actual Triangle	What you *Do/Not Do* in your life to make you *Feel* good about yourself and your life, your future plans. What you *Do/Not Do* that aids you in being with people you like to be with, *Connect,* or *Relate* to people, places, ideas that make you *Happy* or *Satisfied* with your life, help you *Feel* content.
Ideal Triangle	What you *Value,* wish/prefer to *Do/Not Do* to *Feel* good about yourself, your future plans and people/places/ideas you *Feel* part of.
Tailored Triangle	What is more *Realistic* and achievable within a period of time to *Do/Not Do* to aid your *Satisfaction* and *Happiness*.
Congruence/ incongruence	When your current state of life situation and what you *Value*, prefer or wish for are nearly in one direction, there is a *Congruence* and when they fall apart and take different directions, therefore, there is an *Incongruence* in your acts and *Needs*.
Harmony/ Disharmony	If what you *Do/Not Do* to meet one *Need* aids with others, it is called *Harmony*. When your acts to meet one of your *Needs* distances you from the other, or even goes against meeting the other *Need*, it is called *Disharmony*.
Skewed Triangle	When what you *Do/Not Do Satisfies* one or two of your *Needs* only in an exaggerated manner and denies the others, it is called *Skew* and results in a *Skewed Triangle* shape.
Contextual positive	Elements around you that help you to *Do/Not Do* things that are in your favour.
Contextual negative	Elements around you that don't help and may even work against what you *Do/Not Do*.
Changeability	When factors that you consider as contributing to your life are thought to have potential for *Change* and are not fixed.
Coping	When you face *Unchangeable* situations and you need to accept and find a way to deal with them as they are.
Obligation	Elements in yourself or your *Context* that are either not *Changeable* or your *Changing* them requires a lot of investment such that you may find it impossible or extremely difficult to *Change*.
Choice-Making	A decision-making process that starts with identifying what the options are to *Choose* from.
Negative/positive *Assignment* of *Meaning* or *Meaning-Making*	The way you explain an event, act or situation that may provoke a positive or negative *Feeling* in yourself.
Attributing Value	The way you evaluate an event, act or situation as either worthwhile or opposite, your own point of view in terms of the quality or features of something.

The first step in phase II is to evaluate the helpee's *Awareness* of their own *Actual* and *Ideal Triangles* for *Doings*. There are three steps in phase II and the step that the helpee is at can be discerned by evaluating their *Readiness* for *Change*. To facilitate the process of evaluating the helpee's *Readiness*, a mutual understanding of the model needs to be established: working knowledge of the *MOW* principles and terminology in the very early stages of interviewing the helpees is essential. Table 6.1 presents the lay language used for communicating the concepts of the *MOW* with the helpees. Figure 6.1 demonstrates the Decision–Making Chart that guides the steps of the intervention process.

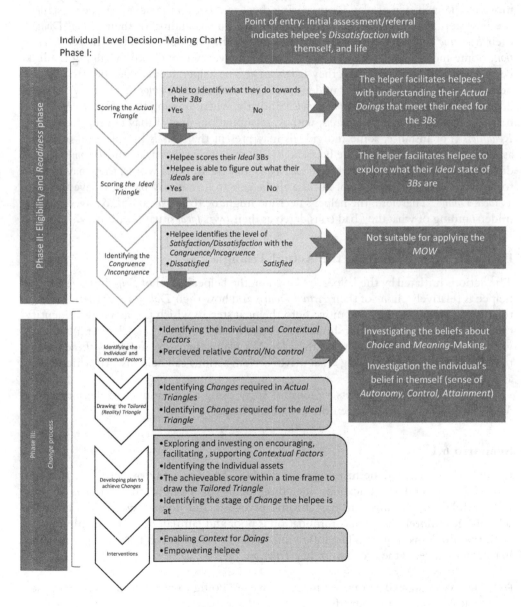

Figure 6.1 Individual Intervention Decision–Making Chart

Some people are not mindful of what they *Do/Not Do* in their life. Moreover, individuals may not be mindful of how their *Doings* link to their sense of *Being, Belonging* and *Becoming*. People also may not be *Aware* of the role that their *Context* plays in shaping and leading their *Doings*. Furthermore, they may lack *Awareness* of the *Meaning* and *Value* they *Attribute* to certain actions or events. Many helpees are not clear about what their *Ideals* literally are. Many of the helpees the author worked with had not reflected on their *Ideals* since childhood, various of their *Ideals* were reliant on things they had been told by others while some *Ideals* had been pushed onto them by their *Context*. Therefore, there is a need to evaluate the helpee's *Readiness* at each step of every phase in order to make a decision to move to the next step or plan for preparing them to move to the next step. For instance, the first step in phase II is clarifying the helpee's understanding of their *Actual Doings*, their *Meaning* and the way they meet their *Needs* at the point of the helper-helpee *Interaction*. Some individuals have a concept about themselves without acknowledging the link between who they are and what they *Do/Not Do*. The helper needs to decide if the helpee needs to be prepared for deeper understanding of their *Actual Doings* or can move to Step 2 that entails drawing their *Ideal Triangle*. Similarly, when drawing their *Ideal Triangle*, the helpee's *Awareness* about their *Ideals,* wishes and aspirations may or may not represent their *Readiness*. For instance, some individuals may present their *Ideals* by speaking of vague aspirations. Others may indicate how they *Want* their *Being, Belonging* and *Becoming* to be different without stating what their *Ideal Doings* may be. In other words, they may be able to draw an *Ideal Triangle* but not necessarily be able to link it to what they have in mind as *Ideal Doings*. Therefore, the helper's decision might be to *Prepare* them to have a clearer understanding of what they had considered as their own *Ideal* situation till now.

Phase II, Step 1: creating the Actual Triangle

The actions initiated by the helper are based on the helpee's level of *Self-Awareness*. If the helpee is relatively *Aware* of their *Actual Doings* and how their *Doings* meet their *Needs* in relation to their *3Bs,* they can move onto the next step in which the helpee can identify their *Ideal Triangle*. The helper should use professional strategies (see Chapter 3) to work with the helpee and explore what they *Do/Not Do* in their life and what these *Doings* may *Mean* to them. Identifying what drives certain actions can help discern which *Needs* are being met.

Below, Scenario 6.1 presents a modified story using a pseudonym to demonstrate a *MOW*-based *Interaction* between the helper and helpee.

Scenario 6.1

Jamilah, 37, is a Bangladeshi refugee in the UK. She has a thyroid problem that has caused her several complications including being overweight that has led to low self-confidence. Her husband has chronic psychosis and doesn't work. She has four school-age children. Their accommodation is poor and Jamilah finds it difficult to cope with the problems at home. The following verbatim conversation between Jamilah and her helper concerns the creation of her *Triangles*.

HELPER: As we agreed in our last meeting, we are going to create your *Triangles* to see what is going on in your life.
HELPEE: Sure.

The helper has explained the idea of *Triangles* and the philosophy of the *MOW* to Jamilah in previous sessions. Now they are going to create Jamilah's *Triangles* together. The helper draws a theoretical *Triangle*.

HELPER: OK, Jamilah now we are going to look at your *Doings* to see how you are meeting your *Being, Belonging* and *Becoming Needs*. So, let's start with your *Actual Triangle* and with the *Being*. Tell me what you *Do/Not Do* in your day to day life for yourself?

HELPEE: For myself... well, I come to [the] refugee centre...but nothing else really...

HELPER: So you mean the time you spend in [the] refugee centre is the only time to *Do* something for your own sake?

HELPEE: I can't *Think* of anything else, all I *Do* is to cook for my children that I hate *Doing* it, I hate cooking, I clean the house which is a waste of time as the house condition is too bad and it never looks fine and I like to escape it as much as possible. I have to take care of my husband as he is not able to take care of himself...by the way, I have several plants at home in our backyard that I take care of them too. I love *Doing* that.

HELPER: Does that mean you take care of plants for your own *Satisfaction*?

HELPEE: Yes, absolutely, I *Feel Happy* when I water them, I even talk to them at times. It reminds me of my own country.

HELPER: Great to see there is something else that you *Do* for your own sake. Let's think more...

The conversation continues and other activities that Jamilah *Does* for her own *Satisfaction* are uncovered.

HELPER: OK, so if we want to score you in what you *Do/Not Do* for your own *Happiness* and *Well Being*, what would you give yourself from minus ten to plus ten? (see Figure 6.2 Scoring Triangle)

HELPEE: What is minus ten?

HELPER: Look here at this *Triangle* (Helper draws a hypothetical *Triangle*), if you *Think* you do something to help you *Feel* good about yourself and only for your own sake then you can give yourself score from nought to ten. This means if you don't *Do* anything for yourself you need to give a zero score here. Remember, that self-care activities that you do such as cooking for yourself, taking a shower, grooming or shopping for yourself also count as what you *Do* for taking care of yourself. Now, the more things you *Do* the score you can give yourself is higher. For instance you may say I go to different places, learn different things I like or enjoy. If what you *Do* is not helping you *Feel* positive, *Healthy* and good for yourself and/or harming your *Well Being* then it means that your score is minus. For instance you may say I *Don't* eat, *Don't* take care of my hygiene, etc. and literally neglect my own *Health* and *Well Being*. Therefore, your score is negative.

HELPEE: I can't be accurate!

HELPER: There is no wrong or right in scoring yourself, it's a way to help you to review what you *Do/Not Do*, what they *Mean* to you and how they contribute to meeting your needs.

HELPEE: Well, I do neglect myself at times when I *Feel* low but generally speaking I *Think* I would give myself score of two out of ten.

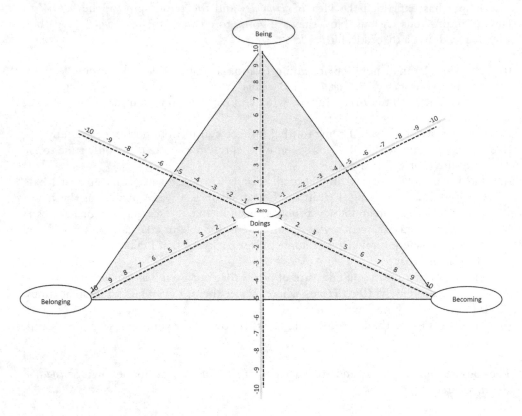

Figure 6.2 Scoring Triangle

HELPER: OK, your guess is good enough, now let's see what your *Doings* are to help with your future plans. Let's start with a near future plan. For instance, what are your plans for the next few weeks?

HELPEE: There is an English class coming up at the refugee centre that is going to start next week. I have told the centre that I would like to attend it.

HELPER: Great, may I ask you to explain the reason for your interest in English class

HELPEE: I would like to read story books in English. I *Feel* embarrassed that I can't communicate with others when there are some community activities. My children feel bad about my inability to communicate with their teachers in parents evening properly so I would like to see myself a mother that they don't feel ashamed of me.

HELPER: You explained your *Becoming* needs very clearly to me, I can see that you see yourself in a near future a person who can communicate more efficiently in English and it gives you a good feeling.

HELPEE: Yes, I wish I could *Do* a lot of things, learn a lot of activities, I love painting …

HELPER: So, again from minus ten to plus ten what score would you give yourself for *Doings* that help you to achieve your aims for your future.

HELPEE: Well, I am not *Doing* much at the moment, I wish I could *Do* more…(pauses) I *Think* I give myself three because I *Don't Do* much really.

HELPER: Fine, so for what you *Do* currently towards your future and who you wish to *Become* you give yourself three out of ten.

HELPEE: Yes.

HELPER: Now let's look at the score you would give yourself for what you *Do* as a member of your family

HELPEE: As a wife I actually *Do* take care of my husband and do almost all of his laundries, cooking, even help him with bathing. Most of my time is spent on cleaning our house and doing house chores for my husband and my children.

HELPER: How *Do* you *Feel* about *Doing* these?

HELPEE: Sometimes, I *Feel* good as my children feel grateful and my husband's family are appreciative of what I *Do*, but there are times I hate *Doing* all these, I *Feel* I am trapped in this situation, it's suffocating…

HELPER: Do you *Feel* that you *Belong* to your family?

HELPEE: I do, and I am happy about it except I *Feel* really lonely as a women left with all these responsibilities and neither can have the support of my man nor can leave him. (Helpee starts weeping.)

HELPER: I am sorry to hear that, it must be really difficult for you especially since/ because that you are away from your own country and family. (Helpee starts crying, The helper gives her a tissue and put her hand on her shoulder.) Helpee continues:

HELPEE: I miss my mother, my home… my heart sinks when I *Think* about there.

HELPER: You look sad Jamilah, I can see how lonely you *Feel* being away from your family on the one hand and on the other not having the relationship you wish for with your husband due to his illness.

HELPEE: Yes, I do…

HELPER: Shall we get back to our task of scoring?

HELPEE: I give minus three to my *Belonging*…I know I have my children here with me but I *Feel* it's me for them and not them for me…do you understand what I mean? I don't like living here…I miss my own country, the nature and the fields I was playing in…The helper uses several empathizing strategies to calm her down.

HELPER: I can feel how upset you have become…would you like to postpone the rest of our task until another time?

HELPEE: Can I go to toilet please and wash my face…I *Think* I will be OK after that…

The helpee, Jamilah, comes back and it seems she feels a bit relieved. The helper continues asking empathetic questions that help them to understand how Jamilah's need for survival led to her marriage and moving out of her own country and how the *Harmony* between her *3Bs* has *Changed*. Jamilah had needed to commit to *Doings* that would ensure a safer life in the country she has moved to but this has led to a separation from her own *Belonging*. Her sense of *Belonging* was more hurt after her husband's mental illness started.

Phase II, Step 2: creating the Ideal Triangle

When an informative *Actual Triangle* of *Doings* is shaped, where significant *Doings* have been noted, the helpee and helper can move onto drawing the *Ideal Triangle*. As mentioned before, the helpee may be *Aware* of their particular *Needs* for *Being, Belonging* and *Becoming* but they may not acknowledge what they may *Need* to *Do/Not Do* to meet these *Needs*. Other helpees may express what their *Ideal* situation may look like through talking about what they wish to *Do/Not Do* yet they may not have *Awareness* of how to meet their *Needs*. The helper's use of strategies to achieve a better understanding of the helpee's *Ideals* is necessary and by extension aids insight when collaboratively drawing an *Ideal Triangle*. In other words, obtaining a clearer picture of the current situation in relation to the helpee's *Triangles* is the core of the intervention. This is done through an evaluation of the helpee's current state to help identify the problems that *Need* to be addressed. Exploring the *Ideal Triangle* with a helpee is a useful process for understanding the helpee's view of themself and their world. It is important to understand the helpee's sense of *Satisfaction* with their life and themself: the *Harmony* they *Feel* within themself and with their life/world. Understanding the helpee's narrative is discussed in Chapter 3.

Phase II, Step 3: analysis of the Incongruence between Actual and Ideal Triangles

The helper needs to explore what the *Congruence* and *Incongruence* between the *Actual* and *Ideal Triangles Mean* to the helpee and how they explain the reasons for the *Gap* between the two, and how *Satisfied/Dissatisfied* the helpee is with it.

   The helper may encounter several levels of *Self-Awareness* amongst the helpees in relation to their *Actual* or *Ideal Triangles* in phases I and II. Below are five likely levels of *Self-Awareness* that the helper may observe:

1   The helpee shows some notion of *Self-Awareness* and is able to score the state of their *Doings* towards their own *Being, Belonging* and *Becoming*.
2   The helpee is not mindful of what they *Do/Not Do* towards their *Being, Belonging* and *Becoming*.
3   The helpee is *Aware* of their *Ideal* situation in relation to wishing to do things differently to meet their *Needs* for *Being, Belonging* and *Becoming*.
4   The helpee is *Unaware* of the relationships between their *Doings* and their *Being, Belonging* and *Becoming*.
5   The helpee is *Aware* of the relationships between their *Doings* and their *Being, Belonging* and *Becoming* but they *Want* to *Do/*Not Do different things to meet them.

Phase III

When the decision has been agreed for the helpee to begin the *Change* process which involves *Re-thinking* and *Re-planning* the helpee's life, the helper explores what the helpee *Thinks* are the factors that hold them back from *Doing/Not Doing* things that aid their *Ideals*. The helpee is invited to *Think* how *Doing/Not Doing* things differently might make them *Happier* and more content with their *Triangles*. The helpee is asked to identify the limiting factors within themself and their *Contexts* that are perceived as contributors to the current *Incongruence*.

   It is useful to consider the ways in which the helper can probe for information about any beliefs the helpee may have that may be holding them back from entering the intervention phase. In other words, looking for *Demotivating* factors is necessary in order to establish whether these factors can be addressed within the helper-helpee interaction or need a more specialized therapeutic intervention that necessitates referral to another service. The next chapter presents the *MOW* strategies to facilitate the process of *Change*.

Having drawn their *Actual* and *Ideal Triangles*, the helpee's views on the *Incongruence* between them are key to the process of *Change* that the helpee and the helper establish together. When individuals perceive the level of *Incongruence* in their *Triangles* as a problem and express that as *Dissatisfaction*, the process of *Change* starts. The individual's beliefs about the perceived benefits of *Change* are the second key point in initiating the process of *Change*. Some helpees might not come to this realization on their own and so the helper needs to facilitate exploration and understanding of the potential problems that the person is experiencing.

Key indicators of a helpee's *Readiness* for *Change* include:

- Feeling *Dissatisfied* with *Self*, life and/or world
- Acknowledging that *Dissatisfaction* may contribute to lower *Well Being*
- Validating the significance of *Satisfaction* with *Self*, life and world as contributors of *Well Being*.

The next chapter presents strategies to initiate the process of *Change*.

It was explained in Chapter 2 that people have different views about the level of *Control* they may have over their life. There are different beliefs about *Choice* versus *Obligation*, the degree of influence an individual may have over their situation and the level of *Control* that factors other than personal characteristics and actions may have on one's life. People refer to a variety of factors that they perceive to be determinants of their actions. Individuals also have different views on the amount of *Change* that they are able to impose on themselves and their lifestyle. Individuals are also different in the way they take *Responsibility* for what happens to them. People's beliefs about their *Choices* and *Responsibilities* therefore indicate how prepared they are for committing themselves to *Change*. As explained earlier in this chapter, intervention could therefore be developed based on the person's *Readiness/Preparedness* for collaborating with the helper to make *Changes*. While *Readiness* refers to the state that a helpee is in at the point of entry, *Preparedness* refers to what happens later when the helper evaluates the potentials in helpee and *Prepare* them to be entered to the *MOW*-based intervention.

The final decision should indicate the next step in developing the intervention *Plan*. In all cases, individual-, community- or society-level aim of the *MOW* is to facilitate the process of *Change*: *Re-thinking and Re-planning* life through *Doings*.

Having taken the decision to enter the individual or group into the *MOW*, there are two main pathways to pursue the *Change process*:

- *Change* in one's views of *Self*, life and the world
- *Change* in *Doings*.

Below is a guide for understanding aspects of an individual's views, beliefs and *Doings* that need to be taken into consideration:

Aspects of an individual's views

Helpees should be able to:

- Find a positive *Meaning* when proceeding with the process of *Change*
- Believe in themself as a *Change-Maker*

- Believe in *Choice-Making* (in perceived *Changeable* factors)
- Believe in their *Capacity* to *Cope with Obligations* (*Unchangeable* factors)
- Believe in their ability to take *Control* over *Individual* and *Contextual Factors*: negative and positive.

Aspects of an individual's *Doings*

Helpees should have:

- Knowledge of what they *Need/Want* to *Do/Not Do* or Capacity of (acquisition) of the related knowledge for *Doings*.
- Skills to facilitate initiation, modification and adjustment for *Doings*.

And be able to:

- *Practice the new Doings* to ensure sustainability.
- *Reflect on the new Doings* to ensure optimum progress.

To *Predict* the outcome of a *Change* process, the helpee and helper should investigate the helpee's personal and *Contextual Capacities*. Through careful evaluation the helper and helpee then draw the Tailored (*Reality*) *Triangle* that indicates what the helpee Expects and hoped for to achieve by the end of the *Change* process.

The following scenario is based on Sarah as a helper who has applied the *MOW* in working with a young person with a learning disability. Sarah (see Chapter 13 for more information) has explored Hannah's *Readiness* and *Prepared* her further to enter a *MOW*-based intervention.

Description and analysis of Sarah's work with Hannah

Hannah is a young girl with whom Sarah has used the *MOW* in helping her to manage several issues that are explained further in this chapter. Hannah has given her consent for her story to be included in this book under her own name.

Sarah's first encounter with her helpee:
    Meeting up with Hannah was made possible through her sister.
    The 17-year-old Hannah gets in touch via smartphone. Some short text messages are exchanged between Sarah the helper and Hannah the helpee to decide on a place to meet.

Sarah's explanation of the *MOW* to Hannah, her helpee:
    Sarah started communicating the terminology and ideas behind the *MOW* with Hannah to see if Hannah finds the *MOW* interesting and understandable and whether she is willing to use it to look at her situation.

Sarah's understanding of her own role:
    In her experience of working with the *MOW*, Sarah perceives herself as a partner being guided by the *MOW* to allow Hannah's inner knowledge to emerge allowing Hannah to become strongly *Aware* of her *Motivations* for *Changing* her situation.

Sarah's *Empowering* approach:

Sarah invites Hannah to choose a place to meet that she enjoys and where she *Feels* comfortable. Sarah *Chooses* her written words on smartphone carefully to support an atmosphere that aids Hannah's *Feeling* that she has been accepted and invited to unfold her stories. Sarah's intention is to encourage a relationship that *Enables* Hannah to open up exploration within herself and her life situation. This *Context* is one that *Enables* Hannah to *Feel* respected and safe during the *MOW* exploratory process. It can be seen here that Sarah has already facilitated a *Context* in which Hannah can present her sense of *Autonomy* and express her sense of *Belonging* to a place in which she *Feels* comfortable, in *Control* and safe.

Hannah *Chooses* a little pastry shop with café that she later mentions is where she works on Sundays as a member of the kitchen staff. On meeting Hannah for the first time in person, it was clear that Sarah's relationship had already been formed with trust and both helper and helpee looked forward to future meetings in person.

Sarah's evaluation of Hannah's *Readiness* to enter a *MOW*-based intervention:

Sarah writes that she sees a young woman, calm and friendly. Hannah shows enthusiasm in the *MOW* exploratory process. This was helpful seeing Hannah's interest in the *MOW* language and terminology and discussing the *MOW* components: *Being, Belonging and Becoming.*

With time, Sarah and Hannah get to know each other and gently unfold Hannah's story through the *MOW* language. When Hannah asked questions about the term *Being,* her body language demonstrated worries and insecurities, her voice changed slightly when asking how to spell/write the *MOW*-related words. She asked if it would be a problem if she did not spell them correctly. Using strategies to *Empower,* Sarah's replies, "This is no problem at all", thereby acknowledging the helpee's worries and reassuring that it doesn't matter if she spells them wrongly and Hannah can always check it with her. Sarah explores Hannah's disquiet and asks her to explain further as to what makes her *Feel* uncomfortable about spelling. Hannah's response demonstrates trust in her relationship with Sarah when Hannah opens up and explains her insecurity and other negative *Feelings* due to her learning disability. Sarah's interpretation of what Hannah says is that her worries lie not in writing difficulties, but in other people's judgements about her which make her uncomfortable. Hannah says that she feels anxious to be not recognized as "stupid" or "less intelligent".

Focus on the sense of *Belonging*:

Sarah describes how, in a later on *MOW* session, she and Hannah discuss the sense of *Belonging* and how it is affected by positive and negative *Meanings*. Hannah explains her low sense of *Connection* with older generations due to the way they perceive gender identity.

Hannah says that,

> In my class, I experience a sense of *Belonging* only to some people. I get along better with the boys than with girls. I like to watch Japanese TV series like animes or chibis. The boys like them too. And I like mangas. I don't *Feel* any sense of *Belonging* and cannot *Relate* to girls' interests in boys, make-up or drinking alcohol, and showing off with vomiting because of drinking too much of it. I even *Felt* like an old woman because of that…quite strange.

Continuing, Hannah explains that,

> Also there are only a few [young] people active in politics. They say... I am just 16 or 17 years old. They vote for the parties their parents voted for. Without even knowing their election manifesto. Or they vote for the party that gives them a present. A pen for example.

Here, Hannah clearly illustrates the ideas and people that she can *Connect* or *Relate* to.

Reflecting on her strong beliefs, Hannah also talked about her family, having their roots in Spanish, Italian and German culture. Her parents met in Argentina where they lived before moving to Germany. She has a brother and an older sister, "She is my idol" Hannah said. Proudly she talked about her family and their environmental *Values* in using as little plastic as possible and almost eating no meat or dairy products.

Within her storytelling, Hannah develops *Self-Awareness* about the people and ideologies she *Feels Connected* to and the *Meaning* and *Value* she *Attributes* to her *Choice* of company. Sarah writes of Hannah's silent pause when summing up *Awareness* of her overall *Feelings* in relation to *Belonging,* when she says, "I spend my time with good people, that make me *Happy*".

Sarah tells that the visualization process involved in drawing Hannah's *Actual Triangle* allowed Hannah and herself to grasp a clear idea of the *Motivators, Facilitators* and *Supporters* as well as the *Inhibitors* of her life situation. There is constant inner movement and *Reflection* visible in the process of silent, confrontation, self-actualization and integration within this space of mutual trust in the *Interaction*.

Helper-helpee *Reflection*:

Sarah writes that before introducing the next step in the intervention, she invites Hannah to focus on how she *Feels* so far in relation to their *Interaction*. With Sarah guiding them through the *MOW,* Hannah is offered another opportunity to *Reflect* on what's happening and integrate possible *Changes* by *Becoming Aware* of them.

Significance of the helper's skills in Interaction and forming the helpee's narrative:

Hannah said that she enjoyed talking to Sarah, because she *Felt* free to express her emotions and *Thoughts* without *Controlling* her words before speaking. She said, "I don't *Feel* forced to do something".

Hannah clearly shows how Sarah's interaction with her that focuses positively on her assets while acknowledging her challenges has established a relationship that has encouraged Hannah to attend the *MOW*-based intervention with Sarah.

When scoring her *Triangles,* Hannah gave herself six for the *Actual Triangle.* She *Felt Motivated* to try and achieve a higher score by working towards greater independence. Hannah's response to Sarah's guidance showed that she was *Motivated* to *Adjust* her *Doings* to achieve a higher score. In an open comment, Hannah said that, "I *Want* to get rid of *Feeling* anxious because of not writing correctly. It is the thought that at my age one should know how to write words correctly". Sarah notices that Hannah is *Self-Aware* about this and that she *Feels* bad about what she considers as her problem, and the *Meaning* that Hannah gives to her inability to spell accurately. Hannah continues by saying, "And I'd like to be brave. I just don't talk to people who I don't know. I need someone to guide me to connect up". Hannah shows interest in *Doing* things differently, to be able to *Connect* to more people. She *Values Connecting* to more people as a strength and the *Meaning* she *Assigns* to this is *Being* Brave!

Sarah and Hannah discuss how to come to a common language that conveys the ideas of the *MOW* to help them to identify where the issues are in Hannah's *Triangles* and how they can draw up a *Tailored Triangle* for Hannah to work towards.

By this point, Sarah notices a *Change* in Hannah's physical appearance and intonation when searching for words. Sarah continues using *Empowering* strategies by encouraging Hannah to take her time to find the words that seem right to her. Sarah finds their *Interaction* moves to a deeper level when they discuss the language of the *MOW* and what it *Means* to Hannah. This process which aimed at *Empowering* Hannah rather than focusing on her weaknesses *Facilitated* the helper-helpee *Interaction* too.

Sarah also observes Hannah's body language while she opens up about her *Feelings* and *Thoughts* about how she *Feels* about herself (her *Being*) and who she would *Value* to *Become* (her *Becoming*). Further, Hannah starts realizing what she *Values Doing* differently in moving towards her Ideal *Being* and *Becoming*. Sarah finds his process helpful in knowing that Hannah is now at a deeper level. This comment of Sarah's is unique as she has *Reflected* on the process of working with Hannah which is the strength Sarah found in their helper-helpee interaction in finding a common language for communicating the *MOW* concepts.

Sarah explains how their helper-helpee sessions changed to become playful, pleasant sessions when searching for the matching translations in the German language and going with the ones that corresponded with Hannah's *Feeling* of *Well Being*.

Sarah notices how a sense of *Belonging* shapes her own *Interaction* with Hannah and conversely how Hannah *Feels* more *Connected* to Sarah as her helper and more committed to the sessions they have together. The relative ease of this relationship helps the move towards identifying the *Incongruence* between Hannah's *Actual* and *Ideal Triangles*. Sarah tells Hannah that she understands Hannah to have a high *Expectation* of herself and using the language of the *MOW* she refers to Hanna's *Ideal Triangle* as needing some *Change* to lower her *Expectation*.

Sarah then guides their *Interaction* towards thinking about a *Tailored Triangle* for Hannah that is more realistic and concise for her near future. Accordingly, Sarah explores Hannah's *Individual Capacities* and positive and negative *Contextual Factors*. Together, they identify the *Changes* required in Hannah's *Doings* by considering the *Changeable* and *Unchangeable* elements of Hannah's *Individual Capacities* and *Context*. When they agree on what is necessary for working towards her *Tailored Triangle*, Hannah smiles when her eyes wander towards the notes she had written *Reflecting* on her *Becoming, saying,* "There will be a lot to come for me".

In turn, Sarah, uses terminology that is understandable for Hannah to identify the *Gaps* between her *Actual* and *Ideal Triangles* so that they can develop her *Tailored Triangle* together. In terms of finding a word for *Incongruence* that Hannah could understand and relate to, the word "match" was used. Hannah was asked to explore it through answering two questions:

1 What is the *Mismatch?* (between the *Actual Triangle* and the *Ideal Triangle?*)
2 What am I doing and what is my aim?

These questions helped Hannah to respond as follows:

1 I draw *(Actual Doing)* instead of studying *(Actual Not Doing)*.
2 I would like to *Do* the laundry *(Ideal Doing)* but I don't know how (Lack of knowledge and skill).
3 I *Do* less than I *Want* (*Incongruence* between *Actual* and *Ideal Doings*), because of the lack of motivation in my school subjects *(Self-Awareness)*.

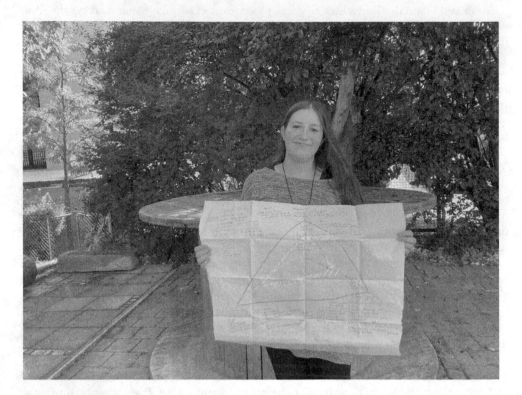

Figure 6.3 Hanna's Triangles

Sarah and Hannah finally agree on what needs to *Change*. They agree that Hannah *Wants* to *Do* a lot which needs to be more *Realistic*; therefore, they agree on more specific and focused *Doings* that will aid Hannah's *Well Being*. They agree that Hannah will *Feel* better if her *Tailored Triangle* includes *Doings* that help her to fill the *Gap* (mismatch) they identified together. Figure 6.3 shows how Sarah and Hannah worked together through the phases and steps of the *MOW*.

The MOW in a public level: assessing needs and evaluating group readiness

While health promotion projects which focus on mental *Health* are in place in some countries such as in Canada, Australia and the UK, *Well Being* through enhancing *Satisfaction* with the *Self*/life on a public level has not been specifically or thoroughly addressed. As such, this is an issue that requires helpers to put forward new initiatives to propose, plan and implement projects to enhance the *Subjective Well Being* of the public, in particular the marginalized and disadvantaged group of people. To start, identifying a common problem that needs to be addressed in the public sphere is necessary such as refugees with a low sense of *Belonging*, children with disability and their sense of Being, Becoming and Belonging. Employing a sociological eye that looks for shared problems among a group of people in a society is a characteristic that a helper interested in working on a public-level project needs to have. Issues raised by professionals like sociologists, psychologists, healthcare services and even politicians could initiate exploration of the matter further. A systematic approach to identifying problems faced by a group of people is needed to avoid unrealistic or misrepresented portrayals. Perhaps, one of the most practical approaches would be to initiate a conversation through networking with other professionals in helper positions. Through networking, helpers should identify a target group with some level of homogeneity. Through identifying characteristics common among a target group, the goal of the project to raise visibility is more achievable. Next, the needs for addressing the problem in the identified target group should be assessed carefully to avoid unsuccessful project plans. The *Well Being* project at a community level is costly, needing much effort to secure a funding and defend the rationale for spending; therefore, investigating factors that help with predicting a positive impact is essential.

The rest of this chapter provides an in-depth explanation of the phases and steps in a *MOW*-based intervention which draws on a real example.

Phase I, Step 1: initial investigation of the *Needs* of the target group

Assessing the need to initiate and invest in a project begins with anecdotal evidence such as concerns raised by individuals or a group of professionals, public authorities and local organizations. Social media coverage of incidents could also offer a point of initial exploration of an issue that may have caused concern.

Identifying a real *Need* for addressing the *Well Being* issues of a target group could be implemented through surveys and focus groups with participants from the group in question, professionals who work with the topic or stakeholders. It is important to investigate the factors that would potentially contribute to the success of or create obstacles for the project. To start with, helpers should look into the existing data about the target group. For instance, helpers may request access to the demographic, social, educational, economic or *Health* profile of the target group.

Phase I, Step 2: identifying resources

Helpers need to look into available databases or their alternatives such as professional bodies, governmental, non-governmental organizations (NGOs) websites and charities to establish potential resources that may facilitate and support the project. In the best case scenario, with a lot of existing supporting factors, developing a *Well Being* promotion project requires financial support. As such, the helpers need to search and secure funds or grants that support the project. Initiating and developing a *Well Being* promotion project is strongly dependent on priorities in governmental budgeting, policies in organizations as well as the local authority's knowledge about and attitudes towards public *Health* and *Well Being*. In some countries like United Kingdom, charities and NGOs are more efficient places to look for resources and financial support. Therefore, helpers should investigate what the best root is for them to take to secure support for their project where they are based at. Figure 6.4 demonstrates the phases and steps when the *MOW* is used in a public level.

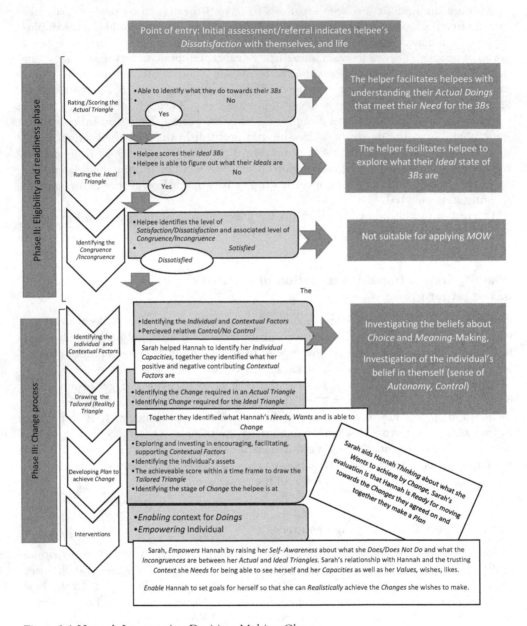

Point of entry: Initial assessment/referral indicates helpee's
Dissatisfaction with themselves, and life

Phase II: Eligibility and readiness phase

Rating /Scoring the *Actual Triangle*
- Able to identify what they do towards their *3Bs*
- No
- Yes

The helper facilitates helpees with understanding their *Actual Doings* that meet their *Need* for the *3Bs*

Rating the *Ideal Triangle*
- Helpee scores their *Ideal 3Bs*
- Helpee is able to figure out what their *Ideals* are
- No
- Yes

The helper facilitates helpee to explore what their *Ideal* state of *3Bs* are

Identifying the *Congruence /Incongruence*
- Helpee identifies the level of *Satisfaction/Dissatisfaction* and associated level of *Congruence/Incongruence*
- Satisfied
- Dissatisfied

Not suitable for applying *MOW*

The

Phase III: Change process

Identifying the *Individual* and *Contextual Factors*
- Identifying the *Individual* and *Contextual Factors*
- Percieved relative *Control/No Control*

Sarah helped Hannah to identify her *Individual Capacities,* together they identified what her positive and negative contributing *Contextual Factors* are

Investigating the beliefs about *Choice* and *Meaning*-Making,

Investigation of the individual's belief in themself (sense of *Autonomy, Control*)

Drawing the *Tailored (Reality) Triangle*
- Identifying the *Change* required in an *Actual Triangle*
- Identifying *Change* required for the *Ideal Triangle*

Together they identified what Hannah's *Needs, Wants* and is able to *Change*

Developing *Plan* to achieve *Change*
- Exploring and investing in encouraging, facilitating, supporting *Contextual Factors*
- Identifying the individual's assets
- The achieveable score within a time frame to draw the *Tailored Triangle*
- Identifying the stage of *Change* the helpee is at

Sarah aids Hannah *Thinking* about what she *Wants* to achieve by *Change,* Sarah's evaluation is that Hannah is *Ready* for moving towards the *Changes* they agreed on and together they make a *Plan*

Interventions
- *Enabling* context for *Doings*
- *Empowering* Individual

Sarah, *Empowers* Hannah by raising her *Self- Awareness* about what she *Does/Does Not Do* and what the *Incongruences* are between her *Actual* and *Ideal Triangles.* Sarah's relationship with Hannah and the trusting *Context* she *Needs* for being able to see herself and her *Capacities* as well as her *Values,* wishes, likes.

Enable Hannah to set goals for herself so that she can *Realistically* achieve the *Changes* she wishes to make.

Figure 6.4 Hanna's Intervention Decision-Making Chart

Phase I, Step 1: exploring, identifying and evaluating the problem through the lens of the MOW

Shared issues that have raised *Dissatisfaction* or *Unhappiness* about a phenomenon in a group of people could be explored using the *MOW*. An example is used to conceptualize a project through a *MOW* filter. As part of a research project investigating the impact of the 2020 COVID-19 measures on students in Britain, the author interviewed a mature student with a 19-year-old son with learning disabilities. The participant explained the difficulties she and other families in the same situation were facing. She mentioned how keeping her son at home had caused her discomfort and dissatisfaction with her life situation. From this interview, an idea emerged about exploring the issues that other families in similar situations were encountering due to the COVID-19 pandemic and isolation/restriction measures. Some of the common issues that the helpee and other families had faced were as follows. Parents and carers found difficulty in explaining the COVID-19 situation to their children with cognitive or mental *Health* issues. They were unable to provide a replacement for activities that suited their children to replace the outdoor activities that they were used to do. Parents and carers were limited in terms of their knowledge and skills to problem solve the issues they were encountering due to government restrictions.

The above list offers an example of a common problem that has been raised by those who have taken on carer roles within their families during COVID-19 measures. From the perspective of the *MOW*, the *Actual Triangle of Doings* had *Changed* for the parents, carers and their children. Due to the unknowns about the COVID-19 pandemic and the uncertainty around the management of the situation by the authorities, the *Ideal Triangle* seemed to have become confused, although parents and carers showed *Awareness* about the impact of uncertainties on their respective *Ideal Triangle*. This example, through the lens of the *MOW*, offers an idea from which a *MOW*-based project could be developed. The identified community group could be the carers of children/with learning disabilities, the aim of the project being enhancement of a sense of *Satisfaction* with the *Self/* life or worlds of those children with learning disabilities and their carers. Identifying a target group that has a problem which can be addressed through the *MOW* does not necessarily mean that the interventions need to be done in a group. However, a group approach to intervention has the usual benefits of the group method. The common principles of group interventions, strategies and leadership skills are employed when running a *MOW*-based group intervention.

Phase I, Step 2: identifying resources

Identifying resources to support a public project depends on the respective country and its systems of *Health*, education and politics, while charities and NGOs are more active in some countries than others. At regional level, politics and socioeconomic factors play the most significant roles in initiating and moving forward *Well Being*-based projects. The most notable element of a project that involves the public and its success in engaging them relies on efficient allocation of supportive resources. Readers (incorrect word) passionate about advocating for such a role for healthcare professionals should explore and lobby for their projects within their countries. This role requires moving beyond the usual boundaries of job descriptions for most individual healthcare professionals in most countries.

Phase II A MOW-based problem identification

This phase can be conducted with the presence of the target group or without them through other methods, including surveys, online calls for stories, photos and paintings. In this section, conducting phase II through creating a group project that brings together the target group is discussed. To start, it is necessary to establish an understanding of what the common problems are and help the target group to identify shared as well as individual ways that they have managed their *Actual Doings*. The above example focused on a problem which emerged as a result of the new conditions of living during the 2020 COVID-19 pandemic. Similar to conducting individual interventions, a group-based project also asks individuals to produce and rescore their own Actual *Triangle*, by identifying what they do to satisfy their senses of *Being, Belonging* and *Becoming*. Unlike the individual intervention decision-making diagram session in which the helpee may progress to the next step or exit to enter a new session, the approach for target groups... you need to finish this sentence. In the group-based intervention session, the aim is to aid helpees in learning more about their *Actual Triangle*. Participants with varying levels of abilities to pinpoint their *Doings* in relation to their *3Bs* help each other in this process. Therefore no one exits from the step-by-step plan. The decision-making diagram is available to show the order of topics that are covered in each step. As such, if the group is not ready, the helper facilitates the group activity to prepare the helpees for doing the tasks required in the current step so that in turn they progress into the next step. Decision making in a group-based intervention is about identifying the time when a group can move or progress to the next step. In other words, the helper is concerned with evaluating whether the group has been prepared appropriately.

Phase II, Step 1: group activities to facilitate understanding the link between Doings and the 3Bs

Activities are used to invite people to *Think* analytically and critically about the common *Doings* that at group-/community-/society-level the target group is engaged with. These common *Doings* link to meet *Being, Belonging* and *Becoming Needs* which are then in turn explored. Asking strategic questions leads to raising *Awareness* about *Doings* and analytically and critically discussing them. Questioning also aids raising *Awareness* about people's *Choices* and *Obligations* at community/society level. It is crucial to remember that projects at a public level aim to educate people, *Enabling* them to learn the *Thinking* process associated with the *MOW* in order to equip them with the knowledge and skills they need to apply the *MOW* at an individual level.

Phase II, Step 2: group activities to facilitate understanding the Ideal Triangle

The main activities in Step 2 are reviewing *Ideal* situations in order to draw *Ideal Triangles*. Individual, community and societal factors that shape the *Ideal Triangles* are explored. The core of this step is to practice asking and answering questions about *Ideal* situations and the potential roots which form those *Ideals*.

Phase II, Step 3: group activities to facilitate identifying the areas of Dissatisfaction and Incongruence

Reaching consensus as to what the areas of *Incongruence* are for the group and for each individual separately are the main tasks of this step. A public-level project is specifically about educating the target group to dig into the roots of *Incongruence*, the *Meaning Assigned Values Attributed* to *Dissatisfaction* and *Incongruence* between the *Actual* and *Ideal Triangles*.

Phase III

All steps explained in the diagram (see Figure 6.5) are similar in nature to what takes place at an individual level. The noteworthy elements of a public-level project concern the way the public is *Motivated* to engage with a *Well Being* project such as the *MOW*. The phases of a public project can be conducted separately and with different purposes. For instance, in phase I, raising public *Awareness* of problems from a *MOW* perspective, among both individuals and authorities, could be a project on its own. Ethically, however, it is necessary to aim for an outcome that guarantees greater *Well Being* than only raising *Awareness* about problems. To raise *Awareness* without providing the required support to manage the problems is likely harmful.

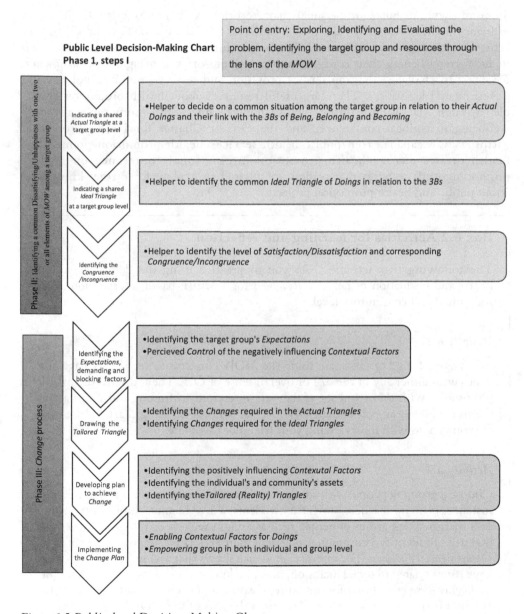

Figure 6.5 Public-level Decision-Making Chart

Helpers' extra skills in developing a public-level project

A healthcare professional becoming an advocate for promoting *Well Being* and mental health at a public level requires several characteristics, what follows are the four main ones:

- Being (incorrect word) passionate? enthusiastic? about public *Well Being*
- Believing that a movement towards *OW* is everyone's right
- Perceiving themself as able to influence public *Well Being*
- Preparedness to challenge authorities.

Some of these attributes are personal characteristics like being eager to facilitate and influence public *Health* and *Value* moving towards *OW* as everyone's right. Others are achievable through educating the helper and training them in required skills which include strengthening their confidence to contribute or even bring about *Change* and *Readiness* to challenge existing service provision and service providers, policies and governmental legislation. There are useful resources about health promotion available through the WHO (https://www.who.int/teams/health-promotion/enhanced-wellbeing/first-global-conference), and the Ottawa Charter for Health Promotion (https://www.canada.ca/en/public-health/services/health-promotion/population-health/ottawa-charter-health-promotion-international-conference-on-health-promotion.html) websites that readers are advised to explore for further knowledge about public and health promotion projects.

Box 6.2 Activities for learning and reflection

The following two activities help you to practice using the decision-making charts and evaluation of helpees' *Readiness* for a *MOW*-based intervention at an individual and community level.

Activity 6.1

Interview a friend or classmate using the *MOW* concepts to see if they have any issues with either any of the *3Bs* or overall sense of *OW*. Then, discuss the *MOW* philosophy with them and see if they are interested in finding out more about themself and any aspects of their *OW*. Use the decision-making chart and see how far you can go with interviewing your friend or classmate.

Activity 6.2

Choose a group of people with similarities in one or more aspects of their life. For instance, primary teachers, university students, a low-income community group, or a marginalized group of people such as asylum seekers or refugees. Look into literature to identify a common problem in their *Well Being*, or any aspects of their *Occupational Wholeness*. For instance, evidence shows that asylum seekers/refugees have issues related to social inclusion, may *Feel* lonely, rejected and lack a sense (or, *Feeling*) of *Belonging*. Look for literature, statistics and even anecdotal evidence for any problem that can be addressed through the lens of the *MOW*.

Summary

Helpee *Readiness* for *Change* was explained in this chapter. A detailed example of an actual *Interaction* between a helper and helpee was presented to demonstrate how a helper may employ their knowledge and skills in evaluating the helpee's *Readiness* and/ or to guide and *Prepare* them for a *MOW*-based intervention. Elements of a group intervention at a public level were briefly explained and supported by diagrams which can be used to compare the similarities and differences between an individual- and public-level *MOW*-based project.

Further Reading

Boyatzis, R. (2006). *Intentional change, volume 25, issue 7: A complexity perspective* (Ser. Intentional change from a complexity perspective, v. 25). Emerald Group Publishing Limited. Retrieved July 22, 2022, from https://public.ebookcentral.proquest.com/choice/publicfullrecord.aspx?p=275495.

Boyatzis, R., & Dhar, U. (2022). Dynamics of the ideal self. *Journal of Management Development, 41*(1), 1–9. https://doi.org/10.1108/JMD-09-2021-0247

Kashdan, T. B., & McKnight, P. E. (2009). Origins of purpose in life: Refining our understanding of a life well lived. *Psihologijske teme, 18*(2), 303–313.

Krebs, P., Norcross, J. C., Nicholson, J. M., & Prochaska, J. O. (2018). Stages of change and psychotherapy outcomes: A review and meta-analysis. *Journal of Clinical Psychology, 74*(11), 1964–1979.

Madsen, S. R., John, C. R., & Miller, D. (2006). Influential factors in individual readiness for change. *Journal of Business & Management, 12*(2), 93–110.

McKay, D. (2021). Motivational interviewing: Accelerating readiness to change. *Journal of Cognitive Psychotherapy*, 35 (2), 87–89.

Norcross, J. C., Cook, D. M., & Fuertes, J. N. (2022). Patient readiness to change: What we know about their stages and processes of change. In J. N. Fuertes (Ed.), *The other side of psychotherapy: Understanding clients' experiences and contributions in treatment* (pp. 73–97). Washington DC: American Psychological Association.

Steger, M., Oishi, S., & Kashdan, T. (2009). Meaning in life across the life span: Levels and correlates of meaning in life from emerging adulthood to older adulthood. *The Journal of Positive Psychology, 4*, 43–52. https://doi.org/10.1080/17439760802303127.

7 Planning the Change

Farzaneh Yazdani

Box 7.1 Chapter aims

This chapter will cover:

- Helper–helpee collaboration in identifying and planning a *MOW*-based intervention
- *Prediction* and *Expectation* as means to aid the *Change* process and *Reflection*
- *Re-thinking* and *Re-planning* processes towards *Change*
- Approaches and methods employed by the *MOW* in the *Change* process

---

Chapter 6 explained how to explore helpees' *Readiness* at every step of each phase and provided strategies to prepare them for initiating the *MOW* intervention plan. Establishing a mutual language and an understanding of the philosophy of the *MOW* is an essential element of *Empowering* helpees throughout the intervention process. The helper, however, needs to evaluate the helpee's situation, cognitively and emotionally, in order to make decisions about the right level of communication in relation to the *MOW* concepts and philosophy.

The *MOW* is used to facilitate an intervention through structuring, guiding and implementing a *Change* process. The intervention consists of employing strategies to make the planned *Change* happen. Regardless of the mode of intervention (individual or group), the helper and helpee collaborate to create a *Tailored Triangle* (*Reality Triangle*) that is *Tailored* to meet the hypothesized optimum possible *Change*. The collaboration happens through *Re-thinking* and *Re-planning* the helpee's *Doings, Thinking, Feeling, Practising* and *Reflecting* processes. *Re-thinking* and *Re-planning* require the helpee and helper to develop a trajectory together. In this chapter, the principles of the *Change* process, namely *Re-thinking and Re-planning,* are discussed. Figure 7.1 shows the *Change* process.

Creating a Tailored (Reality) Triangle

Accepting *Responsibility* for the *Change* process, which includes *Meaning-Making and Choice-Making,* is one of the fundamental principles of the *MOW* which is used to establish the *Tailored Triangle*. While the *MOW* is a *Reality*-oriented model, it does **not** discourage helpees from moving towards their aspirations. According to the *MOW*, it is

DOI: 10.4324/9781003034759-7

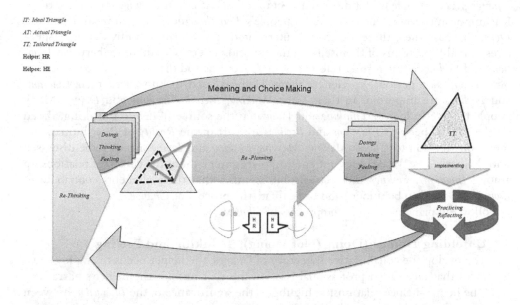

IT: *Ideal Triangle*
AT: *Actual Triangle*
TT: *Tailored Triangle*
Helper: HR
Helpee: HE

Figure 7.1 Change Process

an asset to have aspirations, but it is important that they are not *Unrealistic Expectations.* Therefore, the *Tailored Triangle* is flexible, and its fluctuation allows a person to customize it again and again as and when it is needed. Naturally, *Changes* occur in people's lives and so the *Actual, Reality* and *Tailored Triangles* need to be *Adjusted* according to the person's present situation. It is not only the *Demands* of life that *Change*, individuals *Change* too and the necessity of *Re-thinking* and *Re-planning* is an inevitable characteristic of living. To facilitate the customizing process, it is necessary to indicate the period of time that the *Tailored Triangle* might serve its purpose.

The *Tailored Triangle* has the following characteristics:

- It has significant *Meaning and/or Purpose* which positively *Motivates* the helpee to work towards it
- It is based on the *Choices* made by the helpee
- It is based on the *Responsibilities* of the helpee
- It is based on the *Changeable* factors in the *Individual* and their *Contexts*
- It acknowledges the *Unchangeable* factors related to the individual and their *Contexts*
- It aids the sense of *Being, Belonging and Becoming* through *Doings*
- It facilitates getting one step closer towards a sense of *Occupational Wholeness (OW)*
- It needs to be *Reflected* on when any *Change* happens in the helpee's *Self/Life*
- It needs to be brought to the helpee's attention to raise *Self-Awareness* about *Changes* and their consequences
- It should be used as a tool for *Re-thinking* and *Re-planning* life when needed

Change making: Re-thinking and Re-planning principles

The *MOW* intervention is based on *Re-thinking* one's *Actual* and *Ideal Triangles* and *Re-planning* a *Tailored Triangle* based on in-depth evaluation of the what and how of

Change. Many people find it difficult to get in touch with their *Feelings* at the right time. It is important to raise *Awareness* about people's *Thinking* and *Feeling* in relation to their *Doings* because these three are closely interrelated and inform an individual's perspectives of reality in terms of themself and their world. There is a difference between *Emotions* and *Feelings* as the former refers to bodily reactions and the latter is the presentation of *Emotions* as a person experiences them. Helpees need to know that their *Emotions* and *Feelings* are important in their *Choice-Making*, *Meaning-Making* and *Doings*. Many people believe in logical *Thinking* and *Value* it as the source of decision making. Based on the *MOW*, people's *Emotions* and *Feelings* are part of the *Reality* of *Being* human and their contribution to *Choose-Making*, *Meaning-Making* and *Doings* needs to be discussed with helpees. The *MOW* does not enter into argument about the causative relationship among *Emotions, Feelings* and *Thoughts* but signifies that these elements contribute to *Doings* and need to be understood to facilitate the process of *Change*.

Following principles guide the process of *Change*:

- **Unfolding Doings (Doing/Not Doing), Thinking and Feeling**
  To develop the collaborative trajectory of *Change*, the helper needs to employ strategies that facilitate a professional relationship that unfolds the helpee's narratives. The helper-helpee relationship highlights the significance of the *Interaction* between the helpee and helper in the *MOW*-based intervention.
- **Enabling Practice**
  Practising the planned *Changes* is a way to ensure the sustainability of the *Change*. *Practising* needs to happen in all aspects of the collaborative trajectory: *Doing/Not Doing, Thinking, Feeling, Practising* and *Reflecting*. Commitment to *Practising* needs *Practice* too.
- **Actuating Reflection**
  The act of *Reflecting* on the way a person *Thinks, Feels* and proceeds with the *Change* process is essential based on the *MOW*. Helpers need to educate helpees about *Reflection* as a concept and strategies to implement it in the process of *Change*.

Intended Change

The helper and helpee need to agree on the potential *Changes* that need to take place in the helpee's *Thinking* process: how they view themselves and their world. This is not a simple task, and it should not be perceived as such. The key to managing such a complex task is to break it down and implement it in different steps. Here it is important to look at the different dimensions of the *Being, Belonging* and *Becoming (3Bs)*, and their relation to *Doings* in an individual's *Triangles* as follows:

Change process

Step 1: Re-thinking through Enhancing Self-Awareness and Facilitating Choice-Making

Re-thinking the following:

- **Doings-Being**
In the *Actual Triangle*, a helpee indicates what they *Do/Not Do* to help their *Being*. Before a helper can plan any *Change* in *Doing/Not Doing*, they need to make sure that there is

agreement between both helpee and helper regarding the helpee's *Being Needs*. Table 7.1 shows where the helpee stands in relation to understanding their *Being* needs and their views about their *Ideals*.

When the helpee's views on how to meet their *Needs* for *Happiness* and/or *Satisfaction* are *Unrealistic*, planning *Change* in the *Thinking* processes is necessary. For example, if the helpee believes that they need particular material possessions for their home that are beyond their financial means, this *Expectation* and the *Value Attributed* to it needs to be *Readjusted*; otherwise, it is an *Ideal* situation that is not achievable. Examples of ineffective *Thinking* and *Feeling* that shape the sense of *Being* in connection with *Choice-Making* are:

- *Choices* can be made only if the opportunities are perfect
- *Contextual Factors* are in charge of the *Choices* people make
- People have no *Choice* but are victims of factors over which they have no *Control*
- People are worthy only if they *Do* things with the *Purpose* of accomplishment or achievement in life
- Just to *Be*, enjoying life, and playfulness are not *Valued*
- *Happiness* is only to be found in achievement

- **Doings–Belonging**

There is a need for *Re-thinking* the status of *Doings-Belonging* when people have fixed ideas. For instance, fixed ideas may underpin not only what a good relationship is, but also imbue complex standards for *Being* and *Connections* to others, along with high *Expectations* of *Self* and others regarding *Doings*. *Feeling* guilty, blaming others, over-protection, distancing from other people or places and having a 'must do' rule for themself and others may also feature. Such fixed ideas contrast with more *Balanced* levels of *Belonging* (see Table 7.2).

Table 7.1 Being: Survival, Existing and Living Needs

Needs	*Examples*			
Basic Physiological *Needs* for existing	Food	Shelter	Sexual relationship	Hygiene
Basic Psychological *Needs*	*Autonomy* and *Choice-Making*	*Control* and *Attainment*		
Living *Needs* beyond just existing	*Need* for fun/ playfulness	Rest (*Doing* just to enjoy, *Feel* good)	Not Doing	*Being* alone (free space and time)

Table 7.2 Levels of Belonging

Level of belonging	*Explanation*
Together with others	Sharing places, time.
Related to others	*Relating* through shared things; objects, activities, music, art, food, etc.
Connecting to others	*Connecting* at a deeper level through sharing ideas, values, etc.

• **Doings-Becoming**

Examples of a helpee's ineffective *Thinking* and *Feeling* for being *Satisfied* with themself and their life and/or *Feeling Happy/Well* can be seen below:

• Only a very particular achievement is *Valuable*
• *Feeling* of despair and no hope
• Vision of the future that is heavily based on what others *Think*
• Very high-standard *Idealized* situations that do not seem *Congruent* with the person's *Capacity* and *Contextual* resources
• *Feeling* of guilt, blaming *Self* and others
• Must do beliefs meaning that things must be *Done* in a certain way, and people must behave in a certain way, etc.
• Clichéd *Values* of success
• Exaggerating others' success
• Filtering their own successes and failures by magnifying failures and ignoring/ minimizing successes

Ineffective modes of *Thinking* and *Feeling* are at variance with *Healthy Becoming Needs* (see Table 7.3).

• **Making sense of the overall Triangle of Occupational Wholeness**

Helpers are required to develop in their helpees an understanding of the dimensions of *Being-Becoming* and *Being-Belonging, Belonging-Becoming, Satisfaction* with one's *Self/Life* and world and consequently their sense of *OW.*

It is expected that a relatively *Satisfying (Congruent, Harmonic, Positively Valued and Meaningful)* combination of activities need to be *Done/Not Done* to give an overall sense of *OW.* Linking the helpee's experiences together and bringing them into the helpee's *Self-Awareness* is essential to enhance the sense of contentment and *Satisfaction.*

• Understanding Helpees' views of **Change; Adjust, Modify, Replace or Cope**

A crucial step towards establishing a *Tailored (Reality) Triangle* is recognizing personal factors that cannot *Change* such as personality traits or intelligence and accepting the level of *Autonomy* that an individual can exercise based on these *Unchangeable* factors. Some of these characteristics are easier to identify than others. There are different views on the level of people's ability to make *Changes* to their own characteristics. In today's world, there are perhaps more possibilities for people to *Change* some of their characteristics, for instance physical ones through plastic surgery. The helper and helpee need to discuss what can be considered as *Changeable* within the person. Also, what it takes to be able to achieve that *Change.* Different people may have different ideas on what is considered as *Changeable.* Some individuals consider characteristics,

Table 7.3 Aspects of Becoming Needs

Aspects of becoming needs
Sustaining what is perceived as good/positive, Self-growth, Aspirations, *Planning* for the future, Self-discovery, Instilling hope, Education, *Planning* for achievements, Spirituality.

such as sex, gender, intelligence, skin colour and religion, *Changeable*, while others may see these as *Unchangeable*.

Similarly, an individual's views on the *Changeability* of the elements of their *Context* may be a point for discussion between the helpee and the helper. Elements in the surroundings such as politics or the economy may also be seen as *Changeable* or *Unchangeable*. The helpee may have different views on the extent of *Changeability* and the actions that need to be taken to facilitate *Change* at an individual level or in their *Context*. While the helper's role is not to enter into the depth of the helpee's philosophical views on such matters, the helper is required to challenge the helpee's *Congruence* between what they view as *Changeable* and *Make Choices* accordingly. The helper also needs to ensure that the helpee accepts *Responsibility* for their *Choice-Making*. While it is not up to the helper to try to discuss their views on these matters, the helper is in charge and must raise *Awareness* about the following:

- What is the source of the helpees' views on the *Changeability* of something?
- How does/might this view link to what the helpees *Do/Not Do* and the way they *Feel*?
- How does their view contribute to their sense of *Autonomy*, *Control*, Attainment and their *Feelings* about them?
- How do their views contribute to *Choice-Making* as regards to *Doings*?
- How do their views support or hinder taking *Responsibility* for their *Choices*?

The helper needs to raise the helpee's *Awareness* about the association between their views on the causality of events and their *Doings*. Then, the helper needs to facilitate, support and encourage acceptance to increase the helpee's ability to manage and cope with their *Obligations*. Naturally, what the helper and helpee agree on as *Changeable* leads to the next steps in Intervention. Finally, the helper and helpee need to take actions and commit to *Doing/Not Doing* in the move towards *Change*.

An important point of consideration is the level of distress that the helpee may experience in being exposed to various aspects of their life and their own characteristics and *Capacities* as well as their *Context*. Even for individuals who are very insightful about their own *Self* and world, reviewing their situation/*Context*/past means that they may encounter aspects of *Reality* that most people would find uncomfortable, unpleasant and even traumatic. Giving enough time and using empathy are essential in this matter. Rushing to *Planning Change* can easily lead to an ineffective intervention that can even cause harm. Helpers should give the helpee enough time and space and be *Supportive* when the helpee is going through this revealing process. Helpers may benefit from adopting Compassion-Focused Therapy (CFT) strategies that may aid helpees in coming to peace and further acceptance of themselves and their life. For further details about CFT, you may consider reading an article by Braehler et al. (2013).

The helper then needs to move gradually to encourage the helpee by emphasizing their successes and positive experiences of managing difficult situations in their past and providing feedback on their assets. Helpers need to use several *Empowering* strategies in this step to give helpees a sense of *Control* over the situation and *Enable* them to take *Responsibility* for going through the *Change* process.

Scenario 7.1 is a modified version of a true story which uses a pseudonym. The scenario demonstrates the unfolding of a helpee's story, indicating how the helpee *Assigned Meaning* to her situation and how her views on the situation informed the intervention plan.

Table 7.4 Aspects of Change

Aspects of change	Explanation and examples
Adjusting	*Changing* one or a few aspects of something. For instance, *Adjusting* the level of toilet seats for wheelchair users.
Modifying	Make a particular or minor *Change* in something. For example, *Changing* the time of an activity.
Replacing	*Replacing* one thing for another that is a bigger or more fundamental *Change*. For example, *moving from* a second floor flat to a bungalow.

Scenario 7.1

Sally used to spend time with her grandchildren by taking them to the playground. Since having a stroke, she has been wheelchair bound. The *Doings* in this case relate to Sally taking children to the playground. In Step 1, the helper has facilitated Sally in unfolding the relationships between her *Thinking, Feeling* and *Doings*. Sally is encouraged to *Think* of what it *Meant* for her to take the children to the playground and how she *Felt* about it. Sally mentioned that taking the grandchildren to the playground gave her a sense of *Purpose* for living close to her daughter. She found it positively *Meaningful* to be useful to her daughter, and spending an enjoyable time with her grandchildren gave her a great sense of *Satisfaction* with her life and *Self-Fulfilment*. The helper interpreted taking grandchildren outside as a *Doing* that met Sally's *Needs* for *Being* and *Belonging*. Since her stroke, Sally has not been able to spend time outdoors with the grandchildren. The helper explored how Sally has perceived this *Not Doing*. Sally expressed frustration, and her facial expressions were noticeably sad. The helper probed further into Sally's *Thoughts* and *Feelings*. Together, they agreed that this situation in Sally's life has had a considerable impact on her sense of *Being* and *Belonging*. In her own words, she *Felt* "not useful but a burden".

The impairment due to Sally's stroke could not be amended. While some improvement in her condition has happened due to rehabilitation interventions, Sally still has to live with various limitations and restrictions. The helper explored Sally's *Thoughts* about initiating a *Change* process: how she *Thinks and Feels* about herself, and what she *Thinks* and *Feels* about the role of others in her situation. Sally and the helper came to a mutual understanding about which aspects of her situation could be *Changed*, that is, *Adjusted, Modified* or *Replaced* (see Table 7.4). In the first instance, they discussed aspects of Sally's situation that are difficult or impossible to *Change*: *Adjust, Modify* or *Replace*.

Re-planning

After the first step, where a clear picture of the individual's life and their place within it have been established, the second step begins by developing a hypothesis. A *Predictor* diagram can be made to aid the helpee envisage the outcome of potential *Changes*.

Prediction and Expectation

Prediction is an essential element of *Choice-Making* that needs to be linked to *Expectations*. As part of the planning process, the helpee needs to be clear about what they *Expect* to achieve by *Change* and how they *Predict* the *Change* will affect them (see Figure 7.2).

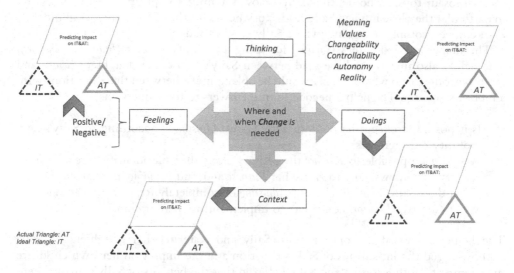

Figure 7.2 Prediction/Expectation Card Board

Table 7.5 A MOW-based Analysis of Sally's *Doings*

Doings-related elements	Analysis/hypothesis
Purpose/Meaning	Spending (cross-generational) family time *Together*, sharing ideas for fun, sharing a sense of joy *Together*, providing free time for Sally's daughter to do other things, being useful and helpful and *Feeling* good.
Procedure	Picking up her grandchildren from their home, playing, having conversations, going to the park cafe, returning her grandchildren home.
Time frame	Twice a week on Monday and Wednesday afternoons.

Step 2: Acting on the plan

Changes in Doing/Not Doing in terms of content, intensity and temporality

Going back to the example of Sally's situation, taking her grandchildren to the playground was a *Doing* interrupted due to a *Change* in Sally's *Health* condition. The helper and Sally discussed Sally's *Thinking* behind her *Doing* (taking grandchildren to the playground). They agreed to investigate further Sally's *Doing* and its links to her *Thinking* and *Feelings*. The helper's analysis of this *Doing* is shown in Table 7.5.

As shown in Table 7.5, Sally had a routine of taking her grandchildren out during the last two years prior to her stroke. She used to walk to her daughter's house to help with preparing her grandchildren for the outing, and then she would take them to the playground for two hours. The helper encouraged Sally to *Think* about the following:

1 What activities would her grandchildren be interested in? (outdoor or indoor)
2 Of those activities, which would Sally *Feel* confident to engage with?

Sally mentioned that her grandchildren, aged four and six years, love to play ball when they are in the playground. At times, they enjoy picnics on the grass in the park with their dinosaur toys. At home, they both enjoy watching TV, playing board games and in particular they love it when Sally reads story books for them. Sally and her grandchildren enjoyed competitive games where Sally acts as a judge.

The helper assessed Sally's *Capacity* for using a mobility scooter (*Individual Factors*). The helper also investigated the road between Sally's house, her daughter's house and the playground as to whether Sally would be able to move between these locations with a mobility scooter. The helper needed to find answers to these questions:

- Is it possible to keep the outdoor activity by *Adjusting* it according to Sally's new mobility requirements?
- Would it be possible to *Replace* the activity altogether and identify a new form of activity that allows Sally to *Attain* her *Purpose* and find *Meaning* in what she *Does*?
- What does Sally *Think/Feel* about *Adjusting* or completely *Replacing* the activity?
- What *Contextual Factors* contribute to implementing these options?

The helper discussed the options with Sally and Katerina, her daughter. Katerina acknowledged the limitations of Sally's situation and the impact on her own childcare management. Both Katerina and Sally believed that the benefits of Sally's involvement in taking care of the children also had a positive impact on Sally's sense of *Well Being*. Maintaining the same level of *Belonging* between Sally and her grandchildren was significant for them. Considering Sally's other symptoms, such as fatigue and occasional poor concentration, the helper suggested options for Sally's *Doing/Not Doing*. Below is what they planned collaboratively:

Adjustment in Doings:

- The time and period of staying outdoors
- Using a mobility scooter to pick up the grandchildren

Replacement for Doing:

- Spending time on an indoor activity instead

To facilitate these plans:

- Sally agreed to discuss the options with her grandchildren and explain the limitations.
- Sally agreed to be educated in the use of a mobility scooter and practice with the helper to *Feel* confident using it.
- Sally accepted that she couldn't play ball in the playground and be actively involved in some of the outdoor activities they used to do together.
- Katerina also agreed to discuss the limitations of the activities Sally can share with her grandchildren and invite them to be more responsible for their own safety in the playground and to limit some activities based on Sally's mobility scooter use.
- There was also a limitation in relation to the places where Sally could go to using her mobility scooter.

After *Planning*, implementation of the plan needs *Practice*. Variety of ways that *Practice* can take place is explained next.

Step 3: Practice

When people repeat what they *Do/Not Do* and the ways in which they *Do/Not Do* them, the patterns are learned by the brain. Repeating patterns of *Doings* is an element of a habituating process. *Temporal* and *Contextual Factors* also contribute to this process. For instance, making tea, the way it's prepared, the time of day at which it's made and the familiar *Context* of an individual's kitchen lead to forming a *Doing* habit. Imagine the first time when an individual is learning how to make tea and all the elements of learning that come together to establish a pattern of tea making. Every step of the activity, how it's *Done,* and its duration, is important to ensure not only the completion of the task but also that it is undertaken in an acceptable manner and that the end product is satisfactory. A breakdown of what is *Done* illustrates the number of steps required for completing the task and the individual's performance *Capacity.* Through practice, the process of making tea becomes more automatic and less cognitively demanding. People develop confidence in *Doing* what they have practised and what is familiar to them. There are, however, two potential problems with habituated *Doings.* Some individuals find it difficult to *Cope* with a situation when the pattern of *Doing* is disrupted for any reason. There are several situations that result in disruption of patterns of *Doing,* some of which are due to natural *Changes* in a person's life when moving from one stage to another. For example, when young people move out of their parental home where they had little *Responsibility* to establish a life that is more independent. In cases like this, individuals are most likely to: repeat the same pattern of *Doing* in the new *Context,* explore new ways of *Doing* and *Modify* previous patterns or develop a completely new pattern of *Doing.* Throughout this process, individuals test and learn about their own *Capacity.* The level of coming out of their habituated pattern, investigating or risking new ways of *Doing* depend on several factors. An individual's personality characteristics, performance *Capacity* level and *Contextual* support or barriers contribute to the extent a person may move from their previous *Doing* patterns.

Disruption in *Doing* may also happen due to illness and *Changes* in a person's performance *Capacity* or in *Contextual Factors.* As discussed above, *Contextual Factors* could be natural life events such as becoming a parent, starting a new job, moving house and so on. On the other hand, there can be more dramatic *Changes* such as the outbreak of war, pandemics or natural disasters. The reason behind disruption to a person's patterns of *Doing* contributes to the way they respond to the disruption. However, in spite of the cause of disruption, the need for learning is an inevitable fact in all cases. The helper, therefore, needs to remind the helpee that the new learning process needs *Practice* to facilitate *Realistic Expectations* and prevent disappointment. It is not unusual for helpers to hear helpees express that their new way of *Doing* has not worked. *Doing, Thinking* and *Feeling* differently need *Practice. Practising* is not limited to new learnings about the way things are *Done, Practising* also impacts on the way a person *Thinks* about their *Doing.* For instance in Sally's scenario, she first needed to *Change* the pattern of taking her grandchildren out by walking to their home, at times running after them playfully. While she was able to manage taking them to the playground and was still able to show her playfulness in different ways, she thought that was not as much fun as for her grandchildren. She couldn't *Feel* the same joy and *Satisfaction* as before. Sally focused on the limitations of the new situation and thought negatively about herself and her performance. This prevented her from experiencing some of the aspects of the new situation which her grandchildren were really enjoying and which she could enjoy too. Repeating the new way of taking her grandchildren out, exploring new ways of being playful and *Attributing* a positive *Value* to the way Sally, her daughter and her grandchildren had *Adapted to* different strategies were all ways to facilitate a new learning experience.

For some individuals, habituation leads to boredom which is associated with a sense of *Dissatisfaction* with a person's *Self* and/or world. When this happens, the individual may need to impose a voluntary disruption in the things they *Do/Not Do* in order to shift towards a more challenging situation.

Therefore, there is a need to plan how *Practising* is going to take place. A graded approach to *Practice* is useful. Grading may refer to a step-by-step increase in complexity of a task, the speed of completing a task, the period of time that needs to stay engaged with a task and the decreased use of support mechanisms such as the presence of the helper and others, along with the use of assistive tools/equipment.

In the context of Sally's scenario, the plan is to start with a session to *Practise* what had been agreed in the presence of the helper. The helper meets Sally at her home where she gets ready and travels on her mobility scooter to pick up her grandchildren. At first, Sally *Practises* using her scooter to navigate the nearby streets, she then completes the route from home to her daughter's house, and from there, continues to the playground where she moves around inside the playground. Next, Sally uses the scooter for meeting her grandchildren to go to the playground.

As the first session requires a lot of attention to follow many instructions, the helper suggested that as a practice round they only go to the playground and come back. The plan for practice continued by increasing both time and elements into the overall activity of going out each session. This is so that Sally and the grandchildren can *Feel* confident.

The next section presents *Reflection,* its significance in a *MOW*-based intervention and the way it should be conducted.

Step 4: Reflect

Similar to all aspects of a *MOW*-based interventions that put an emphasis on the helpee's *Self-Awareness, Reflection,* what it means, how it is done and the way it helps with the process of *Change,* each element should be discussed with the helpee. According to Hatcher and Bringle (1997), *Reflection* is intentional and focuses on an experience for the purpose of learning from it. In the context of the *MOW,* helpees are invited to *Reflect* on what they *Think* about the ways in which they have *Changed* their *Doings* as part of their intervention. Their *Thoughts* on this may relate to how they plan their *Doings* and what it *Means* to them to *Do* things in the new agreed upon way. The helpee is also asked to explore their *Feelings* and bring them into their *Awareness.* It is important that the helper and helpee discuss the relationship between *Thoughts, Feelings* and *Doings.* The helper needs to facilitate the realization of the *Changes* in these three aspects through *Practice.* This is the way that Reflection is implemented within the MOW specifically for the purpose of raising *Awareness* about the *Change* process.

For instance, the plan for Sally was that she used a notebook to write down her *Thoughts* and *Feelings* after her first outdoor activity with the *Adjustments* in place. The elements in Figure 7.2 can be used to guide *Reflection. Reflection* aids to identify if what were *Predicted/Expected* are achieved. Accordingly, the helper and helpee discuss when, where and what has/has not worked and then decide on what needs to be done further as the next action in the intervention.

Approaches and methods to helping

The general approach of a *MOW*-based intervention is coaching. Importantly, a *MOW*-based intervention employs therapeutic and educational approaches as well. Coaching is a process through which a professional helper facilitates improvement to a helpee's life situation (Kamarudin et al., 2020). Within the *MOW*, coaching is demonstrated when helpers guide helpees to explore their *Actual, Ideal* and *Tailored Triangles, Meanings, Values, Choices, Contextual Factors* and *Individual Capacities*. The main role of a helper in a coaching-based approach is to use listening and responding skills to facilitate self-discovery without going into depth concerning likely mental *Health* issues. However, going through a process of *Self-Awareness* requires employing therapeutic approaches that use strategies to manage the situation. Engaging in an exploratory process about *Self* and the world may also bring some emotional issues to the surface that need to be dealt with sensitivity, supported by professional skills. Therefore, having therapeutic skills such as empathetic listening and managing challenging situations such as escalation of anger are essential skills for a *MOW*-oriented helper. An Educational approach is mostly used when, as part of an *Empowering* procedure, the helpee needs to learn new knowledge and skills. In Chapter 8, examples of strategies based on coaching, therapeutic and educational approaches are introduced. A reading list provides resources to enhance knowledge in these areas. Developing skills requires practice.

Within the collaborative process of a *MOW*-based intervention, the helper uses two main helping methods: *Empowering* the individual and *Enabling* the *Context*. The helper needs to use a variety of strategies to assist managing the helping process.

Empowering a helpee is about emphasizing an individual's characteristics, knowledge and skills that contribute to *Thinking, Feeling* and *Doings*. Strategies used may consist of demonstrating trust in a helpee's capacities for *Thinking* and *Re-thinking, Planning* and *Re-planning* and being attentive to and mindful of their *Feelings* not only at the time of *Thinking* and *Doings* but throughout the intervention. *Encouraging* the helpee by reminding them of their strengths in previous experiences is important as is educating helpees about ways of managing and instructing supported by strategies to address their challenges and difficulties. The helper may use strategies to validate feelings and reassure the presence of support to *Empower* the helpee so that they can initiate and maintain engagement with the processes of *Re-thinking* and *Re-planning*. The therapeutic approaches are necessary to ensure this process is as painless as possible. *Enabling* involves identifying and employing facilitating resources, acknowledging the *Context* and encouraging and advocating social support.

Some of these approaches are demonstrated in Sally's story:

Sally was anxious about her grandchildren walking beside her mobility scooter and having to concentrate on child minding and operating the scooter at the same time. The helper acknowledged Sally's *Feeling* (by saying that it's natural to *Feel* anxious as this is the first time you are going to pick up your grandchildren in a different way and by using a scooter). The helper reassured Sally that they could practise the route as a trial (the helper thereby validating Sally's anxious *Feeling* by suggesting that they might look at what they are going to do as an experiment. By calling it a trial, the helper tries to convey that there is no pressure and that they are only testing something out to see if it works) and they can stop if Sally *Feels* overwhelmed at any point (to give *Control* to Sally). These are examples of an *Empowering* interaction. When Sally and her helper arrived at her daughter Katerina's house, the helper asked Sally to review the plan of

---

Box 7.2 Activities for learning and reflection

Reflect on your own knowledge and skills as a help care professional. Which one of the three approaches is more familiar to you, *Coaching, Therapeutic* or *Educational?* What areas do you need to improve your knowledge and skills in?
You may consider reading the following chapters to improve your knowledge of the educational, and therapeutic approaches:

1. Chapter 4 of *Patient education in health and illness (5th ed.),* Rankin, S. H., Stallings, K. D., & London, F. (2005). London: Lippincott Williams & Wilkins.
2. Chapter 8 of *The intentional relationship: Occupational therapy and use of self.* Taylor (2020).

---

the day with the grandchildren (instructing Sally to apply what she has learned as a new plan to facilitate building confidence to *Empower* her).

As part of this exercise, her grandchildren were asked to verbalize what they are expected to do (*Enabling* the *Context* to be facilitative for Sally to put her plan into action). The grandchildren said that they would be attentive to Sally's instructions to slow down, stop at traffic lights and ask how far they can go when in the playground. The grandchildren were also prepared to take responsibility for packing and unpacking the picnic food if they sat on the grass. To take advantage of the situation and make it fun for the grandchildren, Sally brought their attention to how useful the mobility scooter is as they can put their lunch boxes in the back of her scooter. In this illustration, Sally is *Feeling Empowered* as she shows initiative in turning a new experience into something positive by seeing her scooter as an opportunity rather than a limitation (*Positive Meaning-Making* and *Attribution* of *Values*).

Summary

The *Re-thinking* and *Re-planning* processes as the main procedures of the *MOW* for achieving *Change* were explained and illustrated. The *MOW*-based approaches and methods were presented.

The next chapter provides some of the strategies supported by the approaches and methods used in the *MOW.*

Further Reading

Biggs, A., Brough, P., & Drummond, S. (2017). Lazarus and Folkman's psychological stress and coping theory. In C. L. Cooper & J. Campbell Quick (Eds.), *The handbook of stress and health: A guide to research and practice* (1st ed., pp. 349–364). Oxford, John Wiley & Sons Ltd.

Braehler, C., Gumley, A., Harper, J., Wallace, S., Norrie, J., & Gilbert, P. (2013). Exploring change processes in compassion focused therapy in psychosis: Results of a feasibility randomized controlled trial. *British Journal of Clinical Psychology, 52,* 199–214.

Brockbank, A., & McGill, I. (2012). *Facilitating reflective learning: Coaching, mentoring and supervision* (2nd ed.). London: Kogan Page.

Erdös, T., de Haan, E., & Heusinkveld, S. (2021). Coaching: Client factors & contextual dynamics in the change process: A qualitative meta-synthesis. *Coaching: An International Journal of Theory, Research and Practice, 14*(2), 162–183.

Glasser, W. (2000). *Reality therapy in action*. London: HarperCollins Publishers.

Hatcher, J. A., & Bringle, R. G. (1997). Reflection: Bridging the Gap between Service and Learning. *College Teaching, 45*(4), 153–158. https://doi.org/10.1080/87567559709596221.

Kamarudin, M. B., Kamarudin, A., Darmi, R., & Saad, N. (2020). A review of coaching and mentoring theories and models. *International Journal of Academic Research in Progressive Education and Development, 9*(2), 289–298.

Spitzberg, B. H., & Manusov, V. (2021). Attribution theory: Finding good cause in the search for theory. In D.O. Braithwaite & P. Schrodt (Eds.), *Engaging theories in interpersonal communication* (pp. 39–51). Abingdon: Routledge.

Stallman, H. M. (2020). Health theory of coping. *Australian Psychologist, 55*(4), 295–306, https://doi.org/10.1111/ap.12465.

Taylor Renée R. (2020). *The intentional relationship: occupational therapy and use of self* (Second). Philadelphia: F.A. Davis.

8 Implementing the strategies for Change

Farzaneh Yazdani

Box 8.1 Chapter aims

This chapter will cover:

- A variety of activities which can be used at different stages of the *MOW*-based intervention
- Figures and examples to aid helpers in planning and implementing their ˢintervention in collaboration with their helpees
- Interactive helper-helpee exercises to aid the helpee's self-exploration, the *Change* process, Acting on the planned *Change*, Acknowledging/Validating and Monitoring *Feelings*, Developing a *Narrative, Identifying/Adjusting/Modifying* and *Replacing Contextual Factors, Practising* and *Reflection*

Chapter 7 introduced the *Change* process and *Re-thinking* and *Re-planning* principles. The *Change* process presented there consists of four steps. In Chapter 8, strategies and activities are introduced that may be employed by helpers to encourage, *Enable* and actualize the process of making Change.

Self-exploration

Self-exploration of what an individual *Thinks, Feels* and *Does/Does Not Do* can be helped through several strategies for instance those that happen during helper-helpee interactions and those that the helpee acts on in their own time outside helper-helpee meetings. The most significant strategy that is used during an interaction is assisting helpees to transfer their learning about *Thinking, Feeling, Doing/Not Doing* to the outside of the helper-helpee meeting. The helper needs to use skills in facilitating such interaction and employing particular interpersonal characteristics to ensure the effectiveness of the strategies they use. Being compassionate is very important as it *Changes* the entire interaction into a genuine process of problem-solving the issue of knowing what the helpee *Thinks, Feels, Does/Not Does*.

The helpee can be Empowered during the interaction through using the following strategies for self-exploration:

- Probing (The helper seeks more details to explore an aspect of what the helpee has said earlier by asking a question such as You said that you don't like to be part of

DOI: 10.4324/9781003034759-8

your school's gangs as you hate their *Values*, could you explain more about your school's gangs and their *Values*?)

- Clarifying questions (The helper asks the helpee to explain something further to make sure that their own understanding is as close as possible to what the helpee means. For instance, if the helpee says that they had a wonderful time going out with friends to dance festivals, the helper might want to clarify whether enjoyment was based on being with friends or the dance festival itself.)

- *Reflecting* on what the helpee demonstrates verbally and nonverbally (The helper needs to ascertain whether there is *Congruence* or *Incongruence* between the helpee's observed verbal and nonverbal communication. For instance, if the helpee fidgets with their fingers when talking about planning *Change* regarding visiting their father once a week instead of once a month but verbally says: "that's absolutely fine", the helper needs to make sure this change is what the helpee *Thinks* is *Doable* and *Feels* comfortable with. Should the helper receive contradictory verbal and nonverbal messages it needs feeding back to helpee by saying: "I hear you say that making this plan is fine with you, although I sense you *Feel* uncomfortable about it". This non-confrontational *Reflection* aims to bring into the open the helpee's *Feelings* shown by their nonverbal response. The helpee's *Awareness* of incongruence now enables the matter to be discussed further so that *Planning* can be undertaken according to the helpee's abilities and readiness.)

As the helper-helpee interaction should not take a psychotherapeutic direction, the helper should be aware that some of the helpee's verbal and nonverbal behaviour may need in-depth interpretation. Where dominant unseen contributory factors impede interpreting what happens at a helper-helpee meeting, the helper should use strategies to bring the focus of the meeting to what can be explained within the framework of the helper's knowledge and skills. If necessary, the helper should refer the helpee for other relevant therapeutic interventions.

Using the above strategies of probing, clarifying and *Reflecting*, the helper and helpee can decide on *Doing* activities to help them with the process of exploration and *Change*. For each one of these strategies, the helper needs to think about space, time and activity materials (paper, pen, crayons, tablet, clay, etc.) needed for completing the activity and explaining cautions regarding potential sensitive situations that may arise during these activities. Helpers need to practise in advance and be ready for implementing the suggested activity with plans in place in the case of any potential sensitive situation that needs management.

Here are 12 activities to aid with different steps of the *Change* process.

Activity 8.1 Reversing Seats

The reversing seats activity aims to raise a helpee's *Self-Awareness* of the interrelationship between the senses of *Being*, *Belonging* and *Becoming* with *Doing/Not Doing* and contributing *Contextual Factors*.

According to the *MOW*, key factors that underpin *Doing/Not Doing* are the *Meanings Assigned* and the *Values Attributed* by helpees to what they *Do/Not Do*. Chapter 7 explained that developing *Awareness* about the helpee's *Actual*, *Ideal* and *Tailored Triangles* is an essential part of the intervention. To implement the idea of enhancing *Self-Awareness*, the following strategies and activities may be used. After discussing the terminology of the *MOW*, and interviewing the helpee about their *Actual* and *Ideal Triangles*, the helper and helpee reverse role play scenarios whereby the helper becomes a helpee.

Helper and helpee *Change* their seats, and the helpee is encouraged to think of questions about the *Triangles* of the person that the helper pretends to be. The helper can provide a list of questions that the helpee could use in the activity. Through this reversing activity, the helper goes into more detail of what is considered as *Doings* that can meet *Being*, *Belonging* and *Becoming*. Afterwards the helper and helpee return to their original seats and the helper asks questions about the helpee's *Doings* in relation to their *3Bs*. This activity is designed to help *Thinking* differently about *Actual Doings*. The reversing seats activity can be repeated for drawing a helpee's *Ideal Triangle* too.

The helper and helpee can also create cards such as those shown in Figures 8.2–8.7 to stimulate a list of *Doings* in relation to meeting their *Being*, *Belonging* and *Becoming* needs.

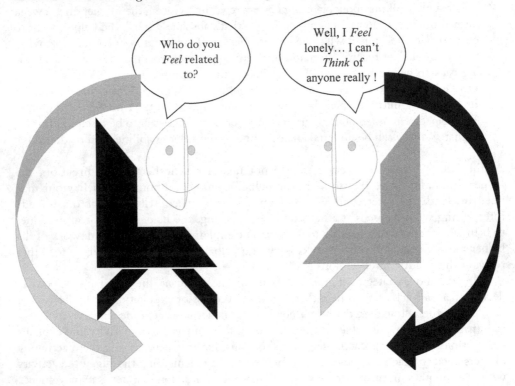

Figure 8.1 Reversing Seats

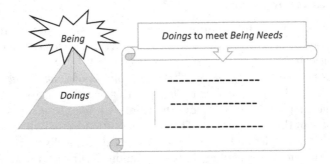

Figure 8.2 Actual Being-Doings

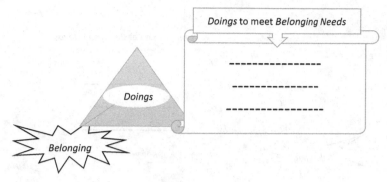

Figure 8.3 Actual Belonging–Doings

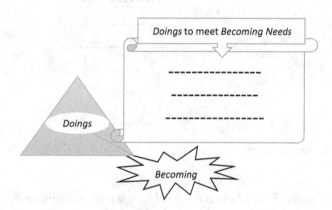

Figure 8.4 Actual Becoming–Doings

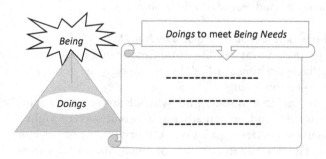

Figure 8.5 Ideal Being–Doings

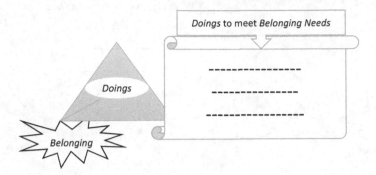

Figure 8.6 Ideal Belonging–Doings

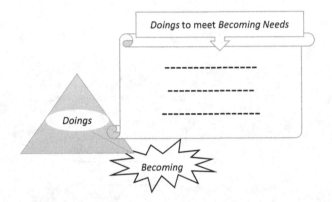

Figure 8.7 Ideal Becoming–Doings

Scenario 8.1 illustrates how Maria and her helper used the reversing seats activity to progress her sense of *Doings*. *The scenario is informed by a real situation but the name is a pseudo name.*
Scenario 8.1
Maria finds it difficult to name *Doings* that help her *3Bs* of *Being, Belonging* and *Becoming*. The helper decides to implement the reversing seats activity to aid Maria's further *Thinking* about her *Doings*. The helper pretends that he is a young man, a university student, who has recently moved to another city and started his higher education course/programme. Their reversed seats dialogue is shown below:

MARIA (M): tell me more about what you *Do/Not Do* that helps with your *Being?*
HELPER IN THE ROLE OF ADAM (A): There are times when I sit on a chair on my balcony and *Do* absolutely nothing as I *Feel* the silence does me good. I just gaze at the garden and get lost in bird song!
M: Oh, so you consider that as something which helps you with your *Being?*
A: Absolutely! I watch stand-up comedy for 10 minutes every night before sleeping to prepare myself for a better night's sleep. Otherwise, my pre-sleeping *Thoughts* make me anxious. This is a way to take care of myself and to aid a worriless sleep.
M: I see … how about what you do for your *Belonging?*

A: I am far from my family, but I *Feel* strong *Belonging* towards them, I am planning to see them during the holiday. I also started developing a social network with my university mates through Facebook.

Maria and the helper *Change* seats and discuss how Maria could *Think* about more things she *Does* that help her *Being* and *Belonging*. The helper presented some examples of *Doings* to aid Maria's *Thinking* about the *MOW* concepts and the indication of *Doings* in day-to-day life that help meeting *Being, Belonging* and *Becoming Needs*.

The next activity presents an idea of *Changing* an aspect of people's *Triangles* that may lead to *Change* in other aspects and through that the helpee learns the link between the *MOW* components and their *Feeling* and *Thinking*.

Activity 8.2 Drawing the Balloon Person

The imaginary balloon person (BP) is used to aid the process of exploring a helpee's situation and to promote *Planning Change*. The rationale behind this activity is that people are mostly more at ease when talking about a third person and potentially staying more logical. The helper draws the BP (see Figure 8.8) and asks questions about how *Change* in the BP can happen and how *Change* in one part may cause *Change* in other parts in BP, and how the BP *Changes* its shape.

Reviewing scenario 1 (Sally), in Chapter 7, the helper can use the BP activity with her and develop a similar situation to Sally that the BP is in and ask Sally to help the BP in managing outdoor activities with their grandchildren after an incident that has left the BP wheelchair bound. Sally can be encouraged to help the BP in the way they *Do, Think* and *Feel* about the situation. Then, Sally is asked to *Reflect* on the *Change*s that

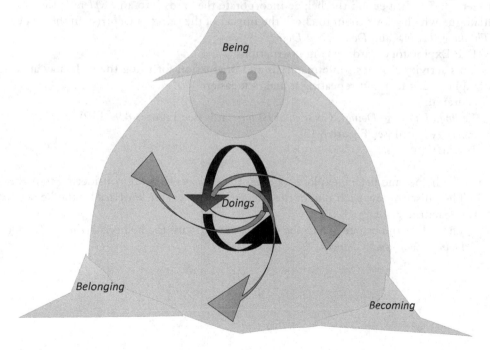

Figure 8.8 The Balloon Person

happen in BP as an outcome of viewing and *Doing* things differently. The helper and Sally then can discuss how the same strategy may apply to Sally.

The next activity is designed to show the interrelationship of the *MOW* components and visualizing the impact of *Changes* on the helpee by breaking down the steps of *Change* with the emphasis on an important factor: *Prediction,* which plays a huge role in *Motivation* and commitment to *Change.*

Going through the Change process

To help people going through the process of *Change,* it is necessary to explore the potential *Changes* that can be made in different components of *Occupational Wholeness* and their potential impacts on other components. People more readily commit to *Change* if their *Expectations* are compatible with their *Individual Capacity* and *Contextual* resources. People's *Prediction* of outcomes of their actions is influenced by their *Expectations. Expectations* refer to the wish to see an outcome of their act or an event. *Prediction,* however, is what they *Think* about achieving their *Expectations.* A helper-helpee collaboration that explores potential *Changes* alongside the helpee's *Expectations* and *Predictions* of those *Changes* and their impact on their *OW* can help to make realistic *Choices.* Activities to help with decision making about what needs to be *Changed* and can be *Changed* are presented in Activities 8.3–8.13.

Activity 8.3 Explore–Predict (E–P) card playing

A set of 16 or more cards with written or pictorial representations of the helpee's *Contextual Factors* is made to be used in this game which the helper and helpee play together. The helper and the helpee incorporate the cards into an *Explore-Predict (E-P)* dialogue which allows them to check the impact of the selected factor(s) on the helpee's *Thinking, Feelings* and *Doings/Not Doings.*

E-P Exploratory Card Playing instructions

This activity requires some materials and instruction for using them. It may appear complicated at first, but repeating it makes it easier.

Material:

Feeling, Thinking, Doings, Contextual Factors cards (see Figures 8.9–8.12)

Activity board (see Figure 8.13)

Instruction:

1   The helper and helpee explore together the *Changes* they are considering to make.
2   They discuss how each one of the suggested *Changes* are *Predicted* by the helpee to impact their 3*Bs.*
3   The helper and helpee add to the cards as they discuss the helpee's *Feeling, Thinking, Doing, Contextual Changes.*

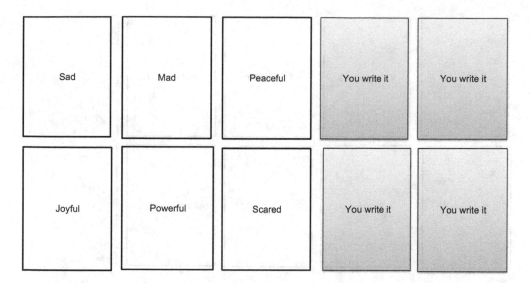

Figure 8.9 Feeling cards

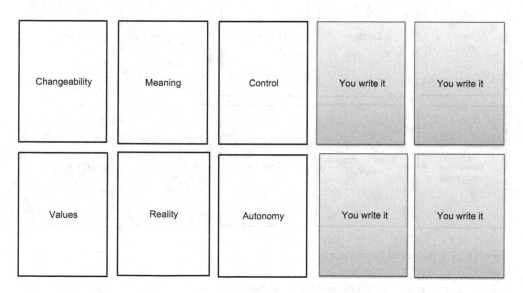

Figure 8.10 Thinking cards

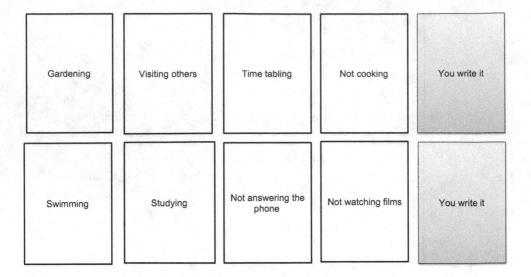

Figure 8.11 Doing cards

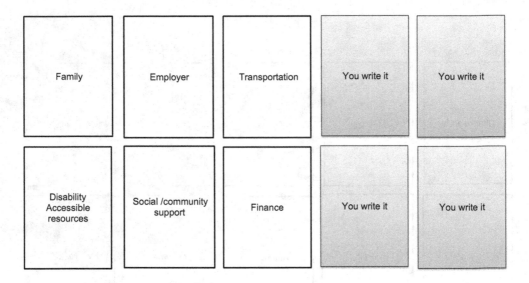

Figure 8.12 Contextual Factors cards

The helper needs to facilitate observation and *Reflection* on the unseen effects of contributing factors to the helpee's situation in forming an experience of *Doings, Thinking, Feeling*. The helper facilitatory strategies encourage the helpee to develop more *Realistic Expectations* of the *Change* process.

The *Change* process can start from discussion of a helpee's *Context, Doings, Feelings* or *Thinking*. If *Change* to the helpee's *Doings* is decided, then its impact on the *3Bs* and the *Context* should be explored and *Predicted*. The suggested *Change* could be in the helpee's *Context* and the impact of that on the helpee's *Doings* and *3Bs*. The *Change* process also

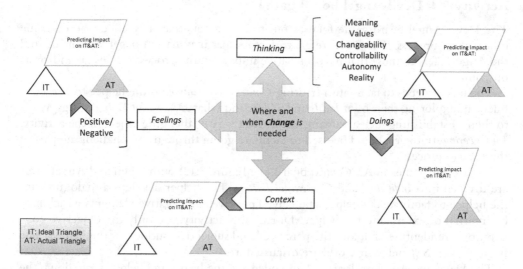

Figure 8.13 Expect–Predict Exploration Card Board

can start from *Thinking* or *Feeling* based on the helper's professional reasoning. The helper also guides whether the impact of the *Change* should be discussed in relation to one or all components of the *3Bs*. The impact of the *Change* should also be discussed in relation to the helpee's *Actual* and *Ideal Triangles*. The *Expect-Predict* diagram from Chapter 7 is used in this game. This diagram can be turned into a board that *Feeling, Thinking, Doings Contex*t cards can be placed.

An example of a *Change* in *Doings* is the activity's starting point presented below.

- The helper and helpee explore potential *Changes* to the helpee's *Doings* which are then written on *Doings* cards.
- They *Predict* the potential impact of each *Change* on the helpee's *Being, Belonging* and *Becoming.*
- They then explore the impact of each suggested *Change* on the helpee's *Context.*
- The *Prediction* of the impact is written on *Predictor* cards.
- When each one of the *E-P* cards has been discussed, the helper and helpee go through a *Choice-Making* and *Meaning-Making* process.
- Together, the helper and helpee continue to eliminate the *E-P* cards that have less significant *Meaning* or low *Values.*
- They retain the *E-P* cards that have more significant *Meaning* and *Values.*
- Finally, the helper and helpee agree on which *Changes* they should *Choose* to work on.

Another outcome of this *E-P* activity, enabled through helper–helpee dialogue, is coming to an agreement about what can/cannot *Change*. The *Unchangeable Factors* should be collected in a *Coping* box (see Figure 8.21).

Through this *Explore-Predict* card playing activity, the helper and helpee can agree upon and work towards the components of a *Tailored Triangle.*

Activity 8.4 Devil-Angel board game

The Devil-Angel board game focuses on unseen factors that may affect the outcome of a *Change* process. The Devil refers to factors that may have a negative impact, and the Angel refers to those that have a positive impact on the process of *Change* and/or its outcome.

The helper needs to facilitate a trusting *Context* that *Empowers* the helpee to *Feel* confident in exploring their own *Ideals* and *Values* and what *Doing/Not Doing* things *Means* to them. Establishing such a trusting *Context* is a very challenging aspect of the activity. *Empowering* strategies should be used to facilitate going through this challenging part of the *Change* process.

To play the game, an A3 *Context* board (see Figure 8.13) with Devil and Angel cards are divided into *Individual* and *Contextual Factors*. The helper develops a dialogue with the helpee to facilitate the helpee's perceived positive and negative elements which may be internal or external to the helpee. During this activity, not only the objective contributors are identified but also the perceived and subjective outlook of the helpee. The helpee's own *Self* and their world are discussed, too.

The Devil and Angel cards are colour coded and the helper and helpee write down the contributing factors on them and add them to the allocated places on the board. The Devil is shown as a snake that bites the helpee and therefore works against helpee's *Doings*. The Angel is shown with a ladder that aids moving forward and implementing the helpee's *Doings*.

The helper and helpee can also use Figure 8.15 to discuss the *Individual Capacities* and *Contextual Factors* that are perceived as *Motivators* for initiating and *Planning Change*.

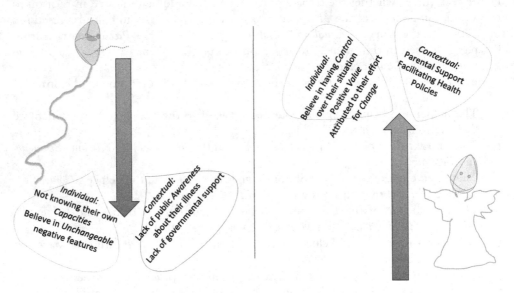

Figure 8.14 Devil-Angel Board

Activity 8.5 What/So-What card sort

In the What/So-What card sort activity, the helper and the helpee identify a list of *Doings/Not Doings* that, if *Changed,* can shift the *Triangles*. The *Changes* may happen in *Actual, Ideal* or both of the *Triangles*. The helper and helpee also create a list of potential

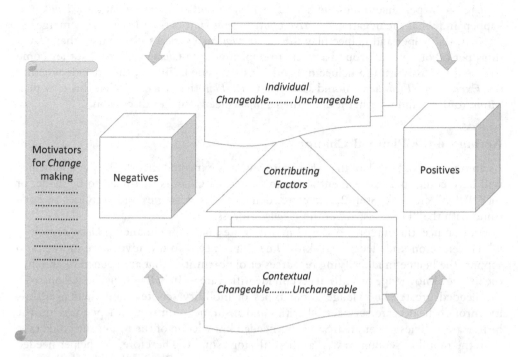

Figure 8.15 Change Motivators

Changes to the helpee's *Context* that *Predict* shifts in the *Triangles*. As discussed in Chapter 7, the *Change* may consist of *Replacement, Modification* or *Adjustment*. The What/So-What activity has different parts to help decision making between *Changing* and *Coping*.

In a What/So-What activity, the helper and helpee come together to create a set of cards based on the helpee's *Doings*. For example, they will identify six *Doings* from the helpee's *Actual Triangle*. They will also create a red, an amber and a green card.

The red, amber and green cards represent the types of *Change* the helpee sees themself being able to make. Red stands for *Coping* without *Change*, amber means making a *Modification* or *Adjustment* while green represents total *Replacement*. The helper presents the helpee with their *Doing* cards one at a time. The helpee is able to put down a red, amber or green card depending on their response to that *Doing* card. With each round of the activity, the helper and helpee discuss: 1. *What* is the type of *Change* planned by the helpee?

2   *So-what* does this *Change* or *Coping* strategy look like?
With each round, the helpee is also able to *Change* the coloured card they have given to *Doings* cards based on their new *Thinking* and *Feeling* about *Doings*.

Each card has space to write what the helpee *Predicts* and *Expects* to happen because of the *Change/Coping* process. Through this What/So-What card sort activity, the helper and helpee develop a dialogue that helps reveal what the helpee *Thinks* about their *Doings*, the purpose of them, what they *Assign* as the *Meaning* of their *Doings*, how they make a link between them and their sense of *Being, Belonging* and *Becoming* and overall sense of *Satisfaction* with themself and the world. When they discuss the *Changes* in

Doings, the helper encourages the helpee to *Think* aloud and share what they *Think* will happen and what the negative/positive contributing factors they *Predict* will emerge.

Next, the helper and helpee play the *Contextual* card sort activity. Then, they plan a short period of time, of around a week, to implement the *Changes*. After that they come back and discuss what the helpee did and what happened. Finally, they decide whether the *Expectations/Predictions* should *Change* and *Re-Plan* the process. What this new plan *Means* to them and whether it helps their *Purpose* needs further discussion.

Acting on the Planned Change

As an outcome of Step 1 of the *Change* process, it is expected that the helper and helpee will have come to an agreement about the potential *Changes* that need to be made, or the "What" element. Step 2, therefore, demonstrates strategies and activities to continue with the "How" aspect of the *Change* process.

For instance, the outcome of Step 1 may indicate a need for enhancing *Doing* capacities which centre on knowledge and skills. The helper needs to use advocative strategies to support the helpee in identifying resources or opportunities that are needed to enhance the helpee's knowledge or skills in certain identified areas. In Sally's scenario (Chapter 7), she needed greater knowledge about types of mobility scooters and their availability through healthcare services, charities and insurance companies depending on the healthcare policies in her area. Sally also needed knowledge of the routes she could take with the mobility scooter as well as the skills for using it. Therefore, the helper needed to use educational strategies to facilitate Sally's learning. To develop the skills, Sally needed to practise and *Reflect* on her learning. As explained in Chapter 7, throughout this educational process the helper employed strategies to *Empower* the helpee.

Acknowledging/validating and monitoring Feelings

Activities to facilitate acknowledgement of *Feelings* and *Emotions* are necessary in an *MOW*-based intervention. The helper needs to use exploring strategies, such as probing and clarifying questions, in addition to projective activities to aid helpees in bringing their *Feelings* to the surface and *Becoming* conscious of them. The helpee should be asked to have a list of feelings and *Emotions* that they can refer to and a good tool for this purpose is Willcox's (1982) feeling wheel (see Figure 8.16).

The helper asks the helpee to identify the *Feelings* and *Emotions* that they can recognize in themselves in general. The helpee is then asked to write down their *Doings* in relation to their *Being* and colour the *Feeling* and *Emotion* components of the figure. They can choose a shade of colour to express the level of negativity or positivity for each of those *Feelings* and *Emotions*.

This feeling wheel can be used to *Reflect* on any aspects of the intervention and at any step of the *Change* process. Shading a new feeling wheel at intervals can be useful in which case the helper should name and date each one of the coloured sheets. The narratives that the helper and helpee create together about what happens to *Feelings* and *Emotions* in relation to *Thinking/Re-thinking* and *Doings*, along with their impact on the helpee's 3Bs, should be written down.

The *Feeling Change* diagram (see Figure 8.17), a simplified version of the feeling wheel, can be used when appropriate. The helper can develop a profile of *Changes* in the helpee's *Feelings* and *Emotions* before, during and immediately after a meeting, to create a visual means for *Reflection* in a follow-up session about implementing the *Change* process.

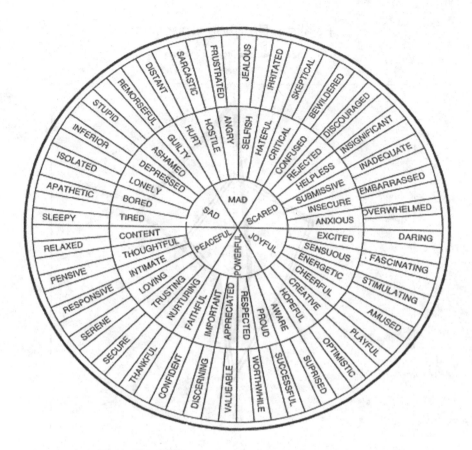

Figure 8.16 The Feeling Wheel. Accessed at https://fosteractionohio.files.wordpress.com/2019/02/feeling-wheel.pdf-FIG_SRC

Each one of the six *Feelings* presented in this simplified diagram is scored between 0 and 10. The scoring can be coloured in each time that it is done for a better visual effect. The scores are then joined to show a shape that represents the helpee's *Feelings* at the time of scoring. This score can be compared with that of previous sessions to discuss *Changes*. Alongside the *Changes* that have been made in any aspects of the helpee's *OW*, the helper and helpee can discuss the link between helpee's *Feelings* and the *Change* and its impact on helpee's sense of *OW*.

Activity 8.5 Picture/film watching

In another activity, the helper and helpee look at pictures and videos and colour or score the feeling wheel and discuss the helpee's *Thinking*. There are examples of pictures that can be used for further exploration of the helpee and their world at the end of this chapter. A professional helper-helpee interaction should facilitate the helper's decision in choosing pictures that could bring out some of the helpee's significant *Feelings* and *Thoughts* in a discussion/meeting.

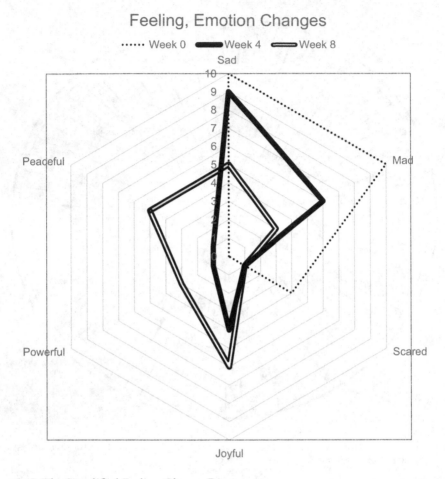

Figure 8.17 The Simplified Feeling Change Diagram

Raising Self-Awareness

Making a link between helpees' *Thinking, Feeling* and *Doings* is key to raise awareness about their *OW.* The three suggested activities which follow are designed to meet this aim: the *Like/Dislike Change*, an imaginary scene and a real encounter activity.

Activity 8.6 Like/Dislike Change activity

The simplified *Feeling Change* diagram (Figure 8.17) can be used when performing this *Like/Dislike Change* activity which raises a helpee's *Self-Awareness* about how their likes and dislikes are connected to their *Doings* which are interrelated to their *Choice* and *Choice-Making.* The activity aids helpers and helpees in *Planning* the agreed *Change.* Showing the findings of the form in a pie chart helps with visualizing the level of *Change* needed (see Figure 8.18).

Like *Doings*	Dislike *Doings*	Need *Change*	From 0-10 how important it is for you to change it 0 not important at all 10 extremely important

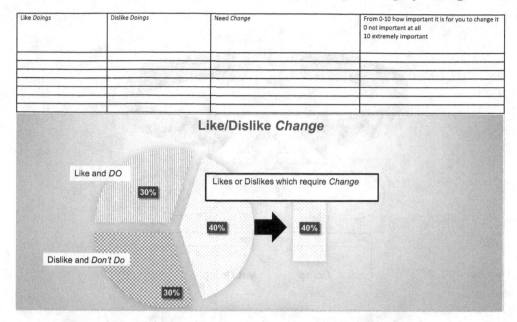

Figure 8.18 Example of a Like/Dislike Change form and Pie Chart

Activity 8.7 Imaginary activity

In the Imaginary Activity, the helper provides an imaginary scene using CDs or online audio stories and invites the helpee to listen, imagine, *Feel* and express their *Feelings* and *Thoughts*. This activity aids making links between the imaginary events and a helpee's *Feelings, Emotions* and *Thoughts* as a means for further discussion about the impact of these *Thoughts* on a helpee's *Choice*-Making and *Meaning-Making* for their *Doings*. A *Doings* chart (see Figure 8.19) is used to aid making these links visible.

Activity 8.8 Real encounter activity

While the helpee is implementing *Changes* in real life, the helper can use the *Doings* chart (Figure 8.19) again to *Reflect* on what is happening in their *Feelings* and *Emotions* having made new *Choices* and *Modified, Adjusted* or *Replaced* their *Doings*. This chart also can be used to *Reflect* on the helpee's *Changes* in their *Thinking* and their impact on *Feelings, Emotions* and *Doings*.

Developing narrative

The *MOW* relies on the narrative created by the helper and helpee about the helpee's *Self* and their life in relation to their *OW*. Creating narratives helps form a *Tailored Triangle* that demonstrates what the helper and helpee plan to achieve through the intervention. Collage Making is a very efficient way of visualizing the outcome of the *Changes* that are planned in the intervention. Any kind of visualizing activity aids getting closer to the reality of the *Change* and its consequences. Below, Scenario 8.2 is used to illustrate the use of collage as an activity in forming the helpee's *Tailored Triangle*.

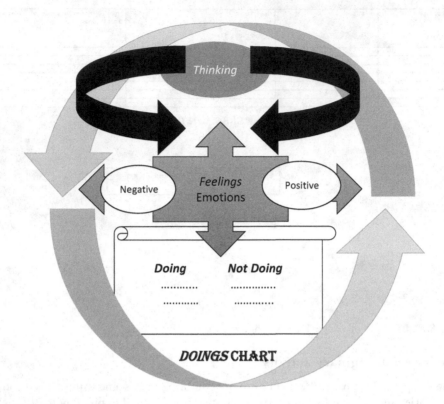

Figure 8.19 Doings chart

Activity 8.9 Collage making

Searching within magazines, cutting out, and sticking pictures on a piece of paper can be used as an activity that helps expression of *Thoughts* and *Feelings*, aids illustrating combinations of *Actual* and *Ideal Doings*, *Meaning-Making* and *Choice-Making*. This activity also facilitates developing the helpee's narrative trajectories.

Scenario 8.2 is a modified version of a helpee's story which uses a pseudonym to illustrate the use of collage as an activity to help develop a *Tailored Triangle*.

Scenario 8.2

Arita is 32 years old. She was studying Mathematics prior to being diagnosed with Major Depression. She finds it difficult to recognize *Meaning* in her life and *Make Choices* to get involved in *Doings*. She is under medication and is currently meeting an *MOW*-based helper. To facilitate the process of *Change* in Arita's life, the helper uses a series of collage activities to engage her with an *MOW*-based intervention. Arita has referred herself and has some motivation to help herself but doesn't know how. Figure 8.20 is an example of Arita's collage making for *Doings* related to *Being* needs design her *Tailored Triangle*. As Arita showed few *Doings* in relation to a positive sense of *Being*, her helper explored her previous interests and habits and reminded her of several potential *Choices* accessible within her *Context* to facilitate her *Choice-Making*. The helper suggested that they might look at some magazine pictures during which Arita was encouraged to recount her memories should she have felt like so *Doing*. The helper paid

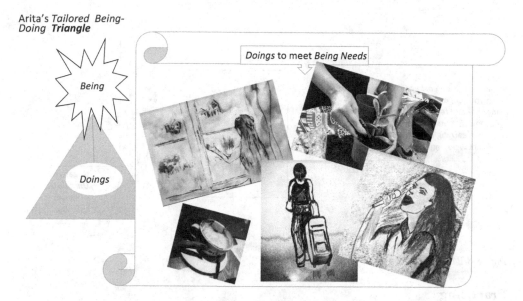

Arita's *Tailored Being-Doing* **Triangle**

Being

Doings

Doings to meet *Being Needs*

Figure 8.20 Doing Chart Arita's Tailored Being-Doing Collage

careful attention to Arita's stories to pick up some of her positive expressions of *Feelings* in what she said or presented nonverbally. The helper checked her *Thinking* and *Feeling* about those options and hypothesized that some of those would likely make a positive difference in her *Sense of Being*.

Identifying/Adjusting/Modifying and Replacing Contextual Factors

In the first step of an *MOW*-based intervention, the helper and helpee discuss the *Contextual Factors* that contribute to the helpee's *Doing*. In the second, third and fourth steps, the intervention is based on what can be *Changed, Adjusted, Modified, Replaced* or *Coped* with. Therefore, the helper needs to establish a collaborative relationship with the helpee using *Empowering* strategies that allow the identification of the *Contextual Factors* and the likelihood of making a *Change* in them. The helper should use *Enabling* strategies to facilitate the process of *Change* to manage the contributing *Contextual Factors* that are perceived as difficult or impossible to *Change*. The helpee also needs to learn and practise ways of *Coping*.

The activities below, insert their titles here, have been created to show ways to implement the *Change* or *Cope* process (see Figure 8.21). It is significant to acknowledge that this process needs to be graded from smaller/less complex to bigger/more complex steps. The following issues need to be discussed between the helper and helpee first:

- Identifying the contributing factors
- Challenging the *Meaning Assigned* to *Doing/Not Doing* and *Contextual Factors*
- Deciding what needs to *Change,* and then *Adjust, Modify* or *Replace* as appropriate, and what needs to be *Coped* with.

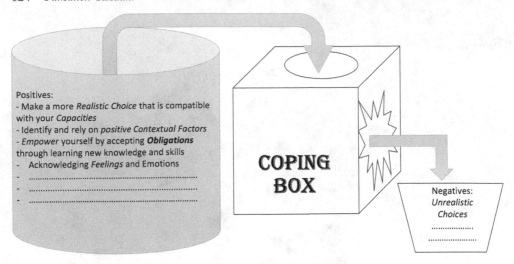

Positives:
- Make a more *Realistic Choice* that is compatible with your *Capacities*
- Identify and rely on *positive Contextual Factors*
- *Empower* yourself by accepting **Obligations** through learning new knowledge and skills
- Acknowledging *Feelings* and Emotions
- ....
- ....
- ....

COPING BOX

Negatives:
Unrealistic Choices
....
....

Figure 8.21 Coping Box

Practising

Practice may happen in different ways. One way to practise is by *Doing* the same things several times. The second level of *Practice*, which is more complex, is to repeat the same *Doing/Not Doing* in the different *Contexts*. The third level of *Practice* is about applying the learnt principles and skills of the prior *Doing/Not Doing* to a new and different pattern of *Doing/Not Doing*. Going back to Sally's example in Chapter 7 to clarify the three levels of *Practice*, in the first level, Sally uses the mobility scooter to pick up her grandchildren for their visit to the playground. Repeating the same path and the same activity is an example of the first level of *Practice*. The second level of *Practice* is to practise using the mobility scooter in day-to-day life and to be able to use different paths and *Doing* different activities.

For instance, Sally could use the mobility scooter to go to the local supermarket to *Do* her weekly shopping. In the second level of *Practice*, Sally *Does* almost the same action(s) but in a different *Context(s),* that is, to progress from taking grandchildren to the playground to shopping in the local supermarket.

The third level of *Practice* is for Sally to use the same principles and skills that she has learned about using a mobility scooter in new types of activities. Sally has learned how to move from her chair to her mobility scooter, how to control the mobility scooter in the street and how to use verbal communication with her grandchildren to keep control of their journey to the playground. In the third level of *Practice*, Sally is set to initiate a totally different activity and uses the same steps of planning and implementation. For instance, Sally *Wanted* to go back to work as a part-time employee, she needed to be driven to her office and she could use an upright walker to move around her workplace. As such she needed to use the same principles and skills she uses when taking her grandchildren out. The helper reviewed with Sally what she had learnt and practised in that activity which could help her in the new activity.

Therefore, the *Practice* plan should be defined between the helper and the helpee following the above levels of *Practice* in relation to any particular *Doing* that needs *Practicing*.

Reflection

It is necessary to identify what the helpee needs to *Reflect* on. As the aim of the *MOW* is *Self-Awareness* about the sense of *Being*, *Belonging* and *Becoming* and overall sense of *OW*, it is therefore essential to evaluate and re-evaluate the helpee's *Thoughts* and *Feelings* in response to any *Change* in their *Doings* or *Contextual Factors*. *Coping* with the things that cannot *Change*, either the helpee's *Doings/Not Doings* or their *Contextual Factors*, has an influence on the helpee's sense of *Being*, *Belonging*, *Becoming* and overall sense of *OW*. It is fundamental to *Reflect* on the impact of *Coping* with *Obligations* and the *Meaning* this has for the helpee. There needs to be *Reflection* on the ways in which *Changes* in *Assigning Meaning* to events and actions would impact on the helpee's *Thinking*, *Feeling* and *Doings*.

Reflection needs to be conducted in relation to *Thinking-Feeling-Doings*. It is an important step of the *Change* process to educate and collaborate with helpees so that they are able to *Reflect* on their intervention. While *Self-Awareness* and the ability to review a helpee's sense of *OW*, *Self-Fulfilment* and *Life Satisfaction*, the main aims of the *MOW* are being able to *Reflect* on the *Change* process that is an essential part of the *MOW*-based intervention. *Change* is an inseparable part of human life and every individual should be able to *Reflect* on what goes on in their life and how it contributes to their *Well Being*. There are several models of *Reflection* proposed for professionals to improve their *Practice*. According to the *MOW*, it is not just the helper but also the helpee who is involved in the process of *Reflection*. The *MOW*-based *Reflection* is inspired by the Borton's (1970) "Model of *Reflection*". The '*What?, So What? Now What?*' approach is adjusted to fit the *MOW* concepts (see Figure 8.22) and is used in collaboration between the helpee and helper to enhance the quality of the *Change* process.

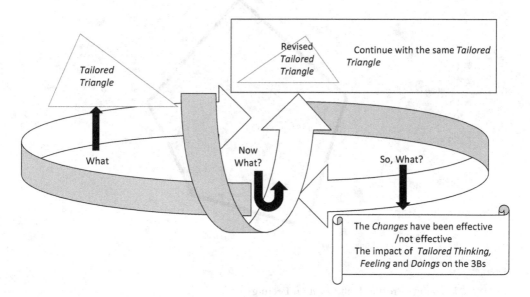

Figure 8.22 What?, So What?, Now What? (3W) Diagram

Activities need to link the person with an internal sense of *Satisfaction* and joy to raise *Awareness* of *Emotional* consequences for *Satisfaction*. Below are some activities for *Reflection* on different aspects of the *Change* process.

Activity 8.10 3W diagram

Using the 3W diagram (see Figure 8.22), the helper and helpee review the *Change* plan to decide on whether they need to alter the *Tailored Triangle*, which *Choices* were made and which proposed *Changes* Worked/Did Not Work and why. The outcome of the *Reflection Practice* should indicate further *Changes* if needed or continuation with confidence.

Activity 8.11 Change profile

Using the *Change* Profile (see Figure 8.23), the helper and helpee can *Reflect* on the impact of *Changes* on a helpee's *Feelings*. The helper and helpee can *Reflect* on how the helpee has been *Feeling* since they agreed and implemented *Changes*. The helpee scores against the *Feelings* identified in the diagram by adding an asterisk (★) sign against it. Then, they join the star signs and it creates a shape that represents the helpee's *Feelings*. This activity can be repeated in different stages of the intervention to help helpee's *Reflection* on the impact of the *Changes* they made on their *Feelings*.

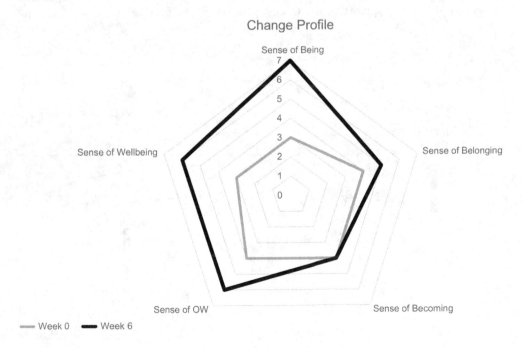

Figure 8.23 Change Profile, Reflection on Feelings

Activity 8.12 Vignette cards

This activity has been created to aid the helpee to raise *Awareness* about the links among *Feeling, Thinking, Doing* and *Not Doing*. The activity consists of three vignette cards and a guide (see Figures 8.24 and 8.25). Each vignette presents a scenario that allows the helpee and helper to discuss the components of the *MOW*. This activity consists of the following steps that can be fully or partially employed based on the helper's professional reasoning:

1   The helpee is encouraged to write or speak about their *Thoughts* on the situation presented in the vignette.
2   The helper needs to use strategic probing and clarifying questions to aid further exploration of the helpee's *Thinking*.
3   The feeling wheel is used to assist illustration of the link between the helpee's *Thinking, Emotions* and *Feelings*.
4   Discuss what the character in the vignette would Do/Not Do and what they would Do/Not Do if they were in the character's shoes.
5   The helper *Empowers* the helpee to explain their *Emotions* and what they mean to them.
6   Next, the helpee is asked to explain how this situation would impact their *Doing* or *Not Doing*.
7   The character's *Prediction, Expectation, Sense of Control* and how they may impact their *Choice, Meaning-Making* and *Doings* are discussed.
8   The role of *Contextual Factors* in relation to the helpee's *Thinking, Feeling* and *Doings* are discussed.

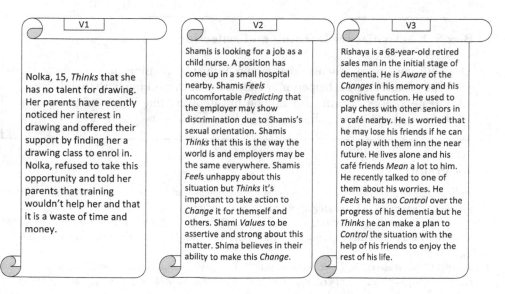

V1

Nolka, 15, *Thinks* that she has no talent for drawing. Her parents have recently noticed her interest in drawing and offered their support by finding her a drawing class to enrol in. Nolka, refused to take this opportunity and told her parents that training wouldn't help her and that it is a waste of time and money.

V2

Shamis is looking for a job as a child nurse. A position has come up in a small hospital nearby. Shamis *Feels* uncomfortable *Predicting* that the employer may show discrimination due to Shamis's sexual orientation. Shamis *Thinks* that this is the way the world is and employers may be the same everywhere. Shamis *Feels* unhappy about this situation but *Thinks* it's important to take action to *Change* it for themself and others. Shami *Values* to be assertive and strong about this matter. Shima believes in their ability to make this *Change*.

V3

Rishaya is a 68-year-old retired sales man in the initial stage of dementia. He is *Aware* of the *Changes* in his memory and his cognitive function. He used to play chess with other seniors in a café nearby. He is worried that he may lose his friends if he can not play with them inn the near future. He lives alone and his café friends *Mean* a lot to him. He recently talked to one of them about his worries. He *Feels* he has no *Control* over the progress of his dementia but he *Thinks* he can make a plan to *Control* the situation with the help of his friends to enjoy the rest of his life.

Figure 8.24 Vignette Cards

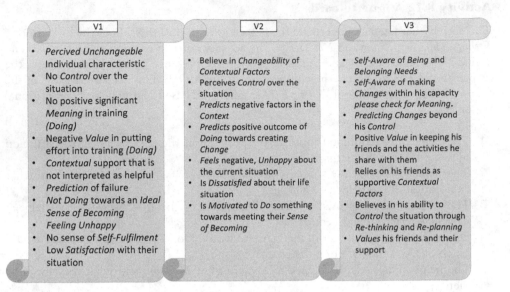

Figure 8.25 Vignette Guide

Summary

Examples of activities were presented in this chapter to aid helpers in communicating with their helpees. These activities can be adjusted and modified based on the helper's professional reasoning. Activities can be used partially according to the purpose of the helper–helpee interaction.

Box 8.2 Activities for learning and reflection

1 With your peers, discuss what factors influence decision making about the type of activities that helpers may choose to use in working with their helpees?
2 Create a series of cards to help you in discussing the variety of *Doings* that helpees may *Choose* to show in their *Actual* or *Ideal Doings*.

Bibliography

Chambers, C., & Ryder, E. (2019). *Supporting compassionate healthcare practice: Understanding the role of resilience, positivity and wellbeing*. Abingdon: Routledge.

Gleeson, N., Parfitt, G., Minshull, C., Bailey, A., & Rees, D. (2008). Influence of surgery and rehabilitation conditioning on psychophysiological fitness. *Journal of Exercise Science and Fitness*, *6*(1), 71–86.

Kashdan, T. B., Barrett, L. F., & McKnight, P. E. (2015). Unpacking emotion differentiation transforming unpleasant experience by perceiving distinctions in negativity. *Current Directions in Psychological Science*, *24*(1), 10–16.

Kirtley, R., & Lister, A. (2022). Adapting recovery through activity for one-to-one sessions. In *Discovery through activity* (pp. 61–65). Abingdon: Routledge.

Lillyman, S., & Merrix, P. (2014). *Portfolios and reflective practice* (Ser. Nursing & health survival guide). Abingdon: Routledge.

Roelke, M. B., Jewell, V. D., & Radomski, M. V. (2022). Return-to-activity: Exploration of occupational therapy in outpatient adult concussion rehabilitation. *OTJR: Occupation, Participation and Health*, 15394492221108649.

Skinner, M., & Mitchell, D. (2016). "What? So What? Now What?": Applying Borton and Rolfe's models of reflexive practice in healthcare contexts. *Health and Social Care Chaplaincy*, *4*(1), 10–19.

Westbrook, D., Kennerley, H., & Kirk, J. (2011). *An introduction to cognitive behaviour therapy: Skills and applications*. London: Sage.

Willcox, G. (1982). The feeling wheel: A tool for expanding awareness of emotions and increasing spontaneity and intimacy. *Transactional Analysis Journal*, *12*(4), 274–276. https://doi.org/10.1177/036215378201200411

9 Reflection as a strategy to enhance Self-Awareness

Farzaneh Yazdani

Box 9.1 Chapter aims

This chapter will cover:

- Two models of *Reflection* that depend on the helper's professional reasoning of the helper–helpee relationship
- Both models which are explained in the context of the *MOW* with examples demonstrating their application

---

Self-Awareness is necessary for initiating *Change* in *MOW*-based interventions. According to the *MOW, Self-Awareness* is essential to initiate a *MOW*-based intervention and is also the outcome of the intervention. Through *Self-Awareness*, helpees can *Re-Think* and *Re-Plan* their *Doings* which strive towards a *Tailored Triangle* that is achievable. This chapter expands on the idea of *Reflection* and how to be a *Reflective* person through *Practising Reflective* writing, drawing and recording during and after a *MOW*-based intervention. *Reflection* applies to both helpers and helpees. This chapter introduces ideas for helper–helpee *Reflective* exercises.

People can *Reflect* on their *Doings, Feelings* and *Thoughts* on different levels. Everyone has the capacity to *Reflect* on different aspects of their *Doings* and *Context* and through *Reflection* improve their situation. The *MOW Empowers* helpees to *Reflect* on their *Actual* and *Ideal Triangles* whenever they *Think* a *Change* has happened in them or their life. Human beings have the capacity to develop and move towards the best of their own capacities: mental, physical and social. The *MOW* facilitates this development for individuals even with very low cognitive capacity. The key to the *Practice* of *Reflection* is developing the right level of *Expectations*. Similar to other aspects of the *MOW* this requires helpees' engagement with the process. *Reflective Practice* requires helpees' commitment. This is important to consider since the level of *Expectation* from a relatively healthy individual, with a high *Individual* and *Contextual* capacity, is different from an individual with cognitive impairments, physical and emotional difficulties and in a *Context* that is inhibiting rather than supporting.

The helper needs to simplify the concepts of the *MOW* and as such the process of *Reflection,* too. Scenarios 9.1–9.3 demonstrate a simplified version of the *MOW* that

DOI: 10.4324/9781003034759-9

can be applied for people with limited *Individual* and/or *Contextual Capacities*. Through these examples, the process of a simplified *Reflection* is explained. Actuating *Reflection* is a step within the *Change* process, as described in Chapter 6, that aids sustainability of the *MOW* which has implications throughout a person's life.

There are several models of *Reflection*. Borton's "Model of *Reflection*" (1970) is explained briefly below with examples of applying the model in a *MOW*-based intervention. In this chapter, the Gibbs model (1988), which is also compatible with the *MOW*, is introduced and explained with examples. In his model, Gibbs explains six steps to help individuals learn from their experience as follows:

- **Description** of the experience
- **Feelings** and *Thoughts* about the experience
- **Evaluation** of the experience, both good and bad
- **Analysis** to make sense of the situation
- **Conclusion** about what the individual learned and what they could have done differently
- **Action plan** for how the individual might deal with similar or more general situations in the future.

Below, each step of the Gibbs model is explained in the context of the *MOW*:

- **Description** of the experience
  The experience here refers to applying what the helper and helpee have agreed on towards making *Change*. The helpee describes an event when they implemented the *Change* plan. This can be a single incident after several implementations of the *Change* plan.
- **Feelings** and *Thoughts* about the experience
  The helpee reports in writing, or by speaking, drawing or recording, their *Feelings* and *Thoughts* during and/or after implementing the *Change* plan.
- **Evaluation** of the experience, both good and bad
  The helpee reports the outcome of implementing the *Change* plan.
- **Analysis** to make sense of the situation
  The helpee needs to review their experience in terms of how, when and where they implemented the plan. How would their *Thoughts* and *Feelings* contribute to the outcome? What and how may their *Contextual Factors* have contributed to the outcome? What are the *Predictors* of the successful/unsuccessful outcome?
- **Conclusion** about what was learned and what could have been done differently.
  Would the helpee need to work on their *Feelings* and *Thoughts*? Do they need to *Change* the time and place of implementing their plan or reconsider/*Change* how they have implemented them? Do they need to explore the *Contextual Factors* in more depth and re-evaluate those *Factors*? And how positively or negatively may those factors have influenced their *Doings*?
- **Action plan** for how similar situations could be dealt with in the future, or general *Changes* that might be found appropriate.
  What does the helpee need to *Change* as a result of the analysis and conclusion? Should the *Tailored Triangle* or strategies to achieve the planned *Change* be revisited?

After implementing and *Practising* strategies to aid *Change*, the helpee and helper need to *Reflect* on the outcome. Effective *Reflection* needs to be concise and focused. The following questions may be useful in guiding the process:

- What are the areas of *Change* that the helpee needed to work on?
- What happened? How did the *Doings Change*? How did the helpee *Feel/Think* about the *Changes*?
- What were the consequences of the *Changes* from the helpee's point of view?
- What are the potential reasons for the successful/unsuccessful outcome?
- Was the success or lack of it on account of the strategies that were used or the way they were implemented? Has the helpee *Practised* them effectively? For how long?
- What *Changes* to the plan/strategies need to be made in order to facilitate success?
- What are the *Predictors* of success? How can new plans/strategies incorporate these *Predictors?*
- What lessons have been learned?

The helper needs to facilitate this exploratory process through asking probing and clarifying questions that help with understanding what has/has not worked according to the plan. *Reflection* should be a collaborative problem-solving approach that leads to further discovery of the helpee's capacities for making *Change*.

Both helper and helpee should *Reflect* on the *Change* process separately as well. For the helpee, this is an exercise to learn the skills that can be transferred to their future implementation of the *MOW*. Helpers need to *Reflect* on their skills in the therapeutic relationships and strategies they applied in understanding the helpee and *Empowering* them through the process of *Change/Reflection*.

Helper–Helpee collaborative Reflection

The helper and helpee can identify a particular aspect of the intervention on which to *Reflect*. This can be suggested by the helpee if they believe there are aspects of their *Plan* that they don't find to work well. Equally, a helper may suggest the time and aspect of the intervention on which to *Reflect*. The point of *Reflection*, however, is not only about problems that have been identified by the helper or helpee. It is valuable to *Reflect* on any aspect of the intervention and bring it into the helpee's *Self-Awareness*.

Helpee's Reflection

It is useful for helpees at Step 2 of Gibbs's model, when *Reflecting* on their *Feelings* and *Thoughts,* to consider what their *Expectations* have been when implementing strategies. What did they expect to happen? How did they *Expect* others to react to them? In the analysis step, it is useful for helpees to check their evaluation of their *Individual* and their *Contextual* capacities. Helpees should *Practise* this process of evaluation with helpers to make sure they can implement it in future on their own.

Helper's Reflection

Helpers also need to *Reflect* on their exploratory journey of understanding helpees and their *Individual* and *Contextual* capacities by asking: Did I explore the components and their relationships effectively? The analysis step for a helper includes questions such as:

- Were my explorations of the helpee's *Individual* and *Contextual* capacities effective in terms of drawing the helpee's *Triangles*?
- Was the *Tailored Triangle* we drew together realistic?

After addressing what may have been the helpee's issue, the action plan should include responses to questions such as:

- Do I need to explore the helpee's situation in relation to any of the *MOW* components in more depth?
- What and how should I discuss the next action with the helpee?

Similar to all other aspects of the *MOW, Reflection* also needs *Practice*. Helpers need to simplify the process for helpees who have lower cognitive capacities and limited *Contextual* support.

A simple process of *Reflection* in such a situation would be to apply Borton's model of *Reflection* (1970) which raises the *3W* questions of *What? So What? Now What?* However, the helper should remember that *Reflection* in a complex situation, particularly so when the helpee's *Individual* capacities are limited which means that the helpee relies more on the helper's direct contribution. Similar to other aspects of the *MOW*, and depending on the *Individual* and *Contextual* capacities of the helpee or the helper, the role of the helper could vary from an encouraging and less directive position to a more instructing and advising role.

The following three examples (Scenarios 9.1–9.3) offer suggestions for applying *Reflection* in *MOW*-based interactions. The scenarios are informed by real cases, and the anonymity of the helpees is preserved through the use of pseudonyms. The *Reflection* process, however, did not happen. Because?

Scenario 9.1

Pietro, a 26-year-old man, has had undiagnosed Attention Deficit Hyperactivity Disorder (ADHD) from childhood. He was forced to leave his country and currently lives as a refugee in a house provided for him and three other refugees. He has been experiencing depression recently, manifested by low appetite, irritable mood and low energy to *Do* his self-care. Others in the house have complained that Pietro has not been contributing to household chores for about six weeks, isolating himself in his room. The refugee service has arranged for Pietro to meet up with a helper. Pietro clearly is *Unhappy* about his situation and *Feels* his time and the energy of youth are wasted, and that he has no future. Although Pietro was *Feeling* down he was still keen to do something about his life. After three meetings between Pietro and the helper, they came up with a plan to help him *Do* things that could help him *Feel* positive about his life while waiting for his political status to be determined and a decision to permit him to stay in the host country. The *Tailored Triangle* they drew together included a couple of activities with several purposes. As Pietro was an athlete and used to *Practise* Martial arts prior to his forced emigration, the helper used his ability as a positive *Meaningful* activity for Pietro to *Do*. From listening to Pietro's story, the helper had realized that being an instructor was more than a job for Pietro as he loved to *Feel Belonged* to a community where he could support young people through his specialism in Martial arts. The helper managed to book a room for him at the refugee centre with a little equipment enabling Pietro to instruct three young male refugees twice a week. By coincidence, two of these three young men were from the same area as Pietro, and in the training sessions, he communicated using their shared first language. Pietro *Felt* that he would not need to know English to communicate with the participants in his class. Pietro had not *Predicted* a situation where there may be other people talking Pietro's native language in his class and conversations may take place that exclude the person who didn't know Pietro's native language. The plan devised by the helper Pietro was to help him *Feel* better about his *Being* by *Doing* exercise and also instructing others. This opportunity was planned to give him a strong sense of *Being* useful. Also, he could *Practise* a little *Autonomy* in class by taking charge of the time between its start and finish and *Planning* what he could *Do* together with his trainees. It was also thought to be a good opportunity to establish a group that he could *Feel Belong* to. However, after five sessions, Pietro seemed to *Feel Unhappy* about the situation, and the helper decided to meet up again and *Reflect* on the plan.

Helper-Helpee collaborative Reflection

Description

The helper asked Pietro to explain what had been happening during the last five sessions, and Pietro gave his account. The helper then asked him to go through his *Feeling*s and *Thoughts* from Session 1. Pietro explained that he was at first so excited and that at the end of the first four training sessions his energy level was better. However, in Session 5, the trainee whom he should have/might have communicated with in English did not come to the class. When Pietro asked about him, the others said that he had mentioned *Feeling* lonely and excluded as the rest could all talk in a shared language that he didn't know.

Feelings and Thoughts

Pietro said that he *Felt* so insensitive and upset with himself. He said: "that was my fault, I should have learned English and communicated with him more often". The helper asked him to look at the experience once again and see how each part of it *Felt*. While Pietro was not very keen to do so, the helper asked him a few questions to facilitate the process of *Reflecting* on the event and Pietro's *Thoughts* and *Feelings*.

HELPER: How was the experience of the other two trainees?
PIETRO: Oh…they loved it, they told me that they *Felt* their time at the training sessions was the best since their arrival in this country.
HELPER: This is nice, how does this make you *Feel*?
PIETRO: I was for a while *Happy* that I could be useful, going back to my routine for exercise and helping others too, like the old days.

Evaluation

The helper continues with exploring Pietro's *Thinking* and *Feeling* about the situation and guides him towards *Thinking* more realistically about the negative and positive aspects of the experience.

HELPER: What does it *Mean* to you to hear they *Feel* good about your training sessions?
PIETRO: Well, actually it *Means* a lot to me. I *Value* what they said about the training sessions.

Analysis

Pietro had not *Predicted* that communicating with all trainees at their training sessions was so important. Pietro *Thought* that he had excluded a member of the group because of a language barrier and was *Feeling* guilty about it. The helper and Pietro *Reflected* on the *Value* that Pietro placed on including all trainees in the training group. In the analysis step of the *Reflection*, the helper guided Pietro to check his evaluation of his own capacity: his willingness to learn English for the sake of his own future in the long term and communicating with his trainee in the current situation. Through this analysis step, the helper explored *Empowering* options for Pietro through learning and *Practising* English on the one hand and looking into *Enabling* his *Context* on the other hand.

Action plan

The helper and Pietro agreed that the action plan would be for Pietro to *Think* about his options for learning and *Practising* English and for the helper to investigate the resources that may be available for Pietro to learn the English language. Pietro also suggested meeting up with the trainee who had left the group to see if he would be interested in looking into options for coming back to the training group. Pietro's intention was to express his willingness to find a way in which they could both *Feel* positive about the experience. As an instructor, it was important for Pietro to show his positive intention (*Meaning* and *Value*) and therefore his immediate action plan was to initiate a meeting with the trainee.

Zara's intervention plan and her *Reflection* is an example of a helpee using the Barton's *What? So What? Now What?* model of *Reflection*.

Scenario 9.2

Zara had a mild stroke about two months ago and during medical investigations, Zara's doctor realized that she is early at the stage of Parkinson's disease. She is confused and scared about her situation. Zara has other *Health* complications and needs to take several medications. She lives alone and her current disorientation and lack of *Control* over her movements has worried her family about Zara's safety at home. She refuses to stay with her children and insists on staying in her own flat. At home, she *Does Not* cook and ignores her personal hygiene, *Feels* lonely and *Does Not* get out of bed. The helper visits her at home. The helper notices that Zara misses her kids/children, *Feels* bored at home and finds herself useless and a weight on her children's shoulders. The helper rationalizes using the *MOW* as she and Zara *Think* Zara has a problem in *Being Happy* with herself, yet missing her children and, therefore, also her sense of *Belonging*. Zara *Does Not Want* to stay with her children, as she *Feels* she is a burden, thus the *Meaning* she *Assigns* to her own presence in her children's life is negative.

Zara needs to *Do* her exercises to help with her movement. She has *Become* so stiff that she cannot move around the house easily. She *Thinks* she is not going to improve and she *Does Not Think* the exercise will help her as she lacks hope and has no *Plan* for the future. Asking the right questions to explore Zara's life assists the helper in identifying that Zara is a great cook, likes dancing and more than anything loves to spend time with her children. The helper's evaluation of Zara's *Context* shows that Zara has a computer tablet but no Wi-Fi at home. Zara's children are *Supportive* and happy to cooperate with the helper in any way that can help Zara. The helper and Zara agree that Zara should *Do* the exercises that her therapist advises through online meetings via WhatsApp and that one of Zara's children should attend each session remotely. Zara was unhopeful that it would help but agreed to *Do* it. Zara *Felt* that meeting her children online would not *Feel* the same and that it would not help with her sense of *Belonging*. Despite her *(Prediction* of ineffectiveness), she agreed to give this a try.

The helper introduced Zara to Barton's *What? So What? Now What?* model of *Reflection*. Through this, the helper meant to facilitate Zara's *Self-Awareness* about the *Choices* she made, the *Changes* in her *Doings* and their consequences for her sense of *Being, Belonging* and *Becoming* and overall *OW*.

Notable *Change* is revealed in Zara's *Reflection* after two weeks.

What?

I have been *Doing* my online exercise for two weeks now. I never *Thought* I could manage it as my legs were too stiff and they used to *Feel* so heavy. I had to learn how to use my computer tablet to get connected to the Internet and call my children. They took turns in reminding me to take my medication. One of them danced with me for 10 minutes a day. I give them instructions on cooking foods the way I *Do*.

So What?

I didn't *Think* I could use the technology but I did. Now, when I look back, I *Feel* glad that I can see my children online. It was unlike what I had *Thought*. It really helped. I wish I could see them in person but I can cope better now. I *Thought* I would never learn anything new anymore and I am going to get older and lose my abilities. Now, looking back at these last few days, I *Think* I still can learn new things and be there for my children. They love my cooking tips.

Now What?

Now that I have realized I can *Do* better than I had *Thought*, I have downloaded two books to read, and am hoping to tell my children what they are about when we meet online. I am *Thinking* of asking my grandson to teach me how to play games on my computer tablet. I *Don't Think* I need my kids to remind me of my medication anymore. I still need to *Practise* using WhatsApp to record my voice and send photos, though.

Zara's *Tailored Triangle* suggests a higher score for *Becoming* as Zara now hopes to achieve new things and progress with the use of technology. Her sense of *Belonging* seems to be more fully met and she expresses *Satisfaction* with her *Belonging* needs. She tries to help herself to *Feel Connected* to her children through sending cooking advice and messages for their birthdays, New Year, etc. Her sense of *Being* has improved and she is trying to achieve a higher score in that by taking more care of herself. She believes through taking care of herself she can make her children happier and less worried. Her self-worth is deeply enmeshed with her children's happiness which the helper has acknowledged in their *Planning*.

Helper's Reflection (Zara's scenario)

What?

Together with Zara, I arranged Wi-Fi for her house, and set up WhatsApp. To *Empower* Zara, I reminded her of the stories she told me about the time she had a car accident a few years back and the way she had had to manage her life, her success in that and her strengths that helped her through that difficult situation. I *Empowered* Zara by educating her in using her computer tablet, Internet and social media. *Enabling* Zara's children to communicate with her online was a big step towards improvement in meeting Zara's *Belonging* needs. Zara was quickly and widely using her access to the Internet for learning, entertainment and finding new stories to tell her children.

So What?

I realized that I had not quite understood the significance of Zara's *Feeling* of self-worth as a mother and the astonishing impact that this had on other aspects of her life. Everything for Zara, all her *Doings,* were linked to the *Meaning* that Zara was *Assigning* to them in association to her children. I had not realized the extent of the impact that Zara's role as a mother and the *Responsibilities* she considered to be hers had on Her overall sense of *Being* and *OW.*

Now What?

Considering the extent to which Zara's sense of *Being, Belonging, Becoming* and overall *OW* had *Changed* through *Doing* anything and everything that could make her more *Connected* to her children, I had to listen more to Zara to learn about any *Doings* that could sustain her positive *Feelings* in the long term. I need to have a more thorough evaluation of what Zara can *Do* and likes to *Do*. Through this, the next step would be: first maintain the level of Zara's engagement with the current *Doings* and, second, plan for Zara to take *Control* over her situation, *Re-thinking* and *Re-planning* for the future.

Strategies to help with Reflection

In Chapter 8, several activities to aid *Reflection* were presented. In this chapter, Scenario 9.3 illustrates how a helper uses writing and note-taking to implement *Reflection.*

Scenario 9.3

Referring back to Sally's scenario in Chapter 7, the helper gave Sally a notebook to write details of her experiences in taking her grandchildren out. At first, Sally was encouraged to just freely write her *Thoughts* and *Feelings*. At subsequent meetings with her helper, Sally's writing was used as a starting point for *Reflection*. Sally wrote that at first her mind was focusing on what she couldn't *Do* and how she *Felt* frustrated because she wasn't able to play the games she used to play with her grandchildren in the park:

> I couldn't hold my grandchildren's hands while moving with the mobility scooter, when I reach the playground, I had to let them go on by themselves…which made

me *Feel* anxious and left with a *Feeling* of being useless...I was frustrated with my inability to walk and not being able to get closer to them while they played... I *Thought* to call them and return home.

The helper illustrated the relationship between the way Sally had interpreted her own *Feeling* of anxiety and *Thinking* herself useless, both of which led to frustration which in turn made Sally *Feel* that she should go back home *(Doing)*. Consequently, Sally's *Feeling* was that she should not take the grandchildren out again *(Not Doing)*. The helper then asked Sally to write about the experience of taking her grandchildren out again and this time focusing on the things she was able to *Do*. For instance, how she managed to get to the playground with her grandchildren walking by her side. To assist Sally in being able to see the positive aspects of the situation, the helper used a probing strategy. The helper asked Sally the following questions:

HELPER: How did you coordinate the speed of your movement on the mobility scooter with the pace of your grandchildren's walking?
SALLY: At first, I was too fast and then I managed to *Control* the speed of the mobility scooter and talked to the grandchildren. I told them to follow my instructions when I asked them to speed up or slow down at certain times.
HELPER: So you were alright in getting to the playground?
SALLY: Oh, yeah I was OK.
HELPER: What did your grandchildren do in the playground?
SALLY: Well, they had a ball and they played with it and then the little one was distracted by a butterfly...he managed to catch and bring it to show me.
HELPER: Seems like he had a good time, right?
SALLY: I *Think* so...
HELPER: Sally, am I right to think that you were taking your grandchildren out to have a good time and provide your daughter with some spare time?
SALLY: Well, yes!
HELPER: It seems to me that this has happened, would you agree?

Sally gradually began to notice that she was still able to *Do* and began to get used to the idea of managing her new situation. She began to *Feel* more positive about herself. She *Felt* that she had been useful through helping her daughter with her childcare. In her journal, Sally mentioned how her sense of *Belonging* had increased as she could see how her daughter and grandchildren enjoyed and *Valued* being around her and how they put effort into making the new arrangements work.

Types of Reflection

Three types of *Reflection* are explained most commonly in textbooks for the purpose of help care profesionals' learning. Healthcare professionals are advised to use all the three when appropriate. *Reflection* on action is concerned with applying the *Reflection* process after an event while *Reflection* in action focuses on applying steps of *Reflection* at the time of an event occurring and modifying the action straight away while the experience is still happening. The third and most frequently advised type of *Reflection* is *Reflection* for action which is used in collaborative helper-helpee interactions. This type of *Reflection* happens after an event but specifically for the purpose of *Prediction* and *Planning* in the context of a *MOW*-based intervention.

Presented below is a brief example of *Reflective Practice* by a *MOW* scholar, Sarah Kufner, on her work with a young girl called Hannah.

The aim here was to *Reflect* on the initial stage of the *MOW* and Hannah's *Readiness* for continuing with the interaction. Sarah introduced Barton's *3W* model by asking a number of questions. To explore and facilitate *Reflection* on Hannah's experience of using the *MOW Triangles*, Sarah asked Hannah the following question to explore *What* has happened.

Please check the sequence and formatting of the dialogue below.

SARAH: How easy was it for you to visualize the process of our interaction? *(What?)*

HANNAH: It was difficult in the beginning because I had no idea what it would lead to and how it would look in the end. But having you guiding me it became simple. (please check that this is Hannah's correct response).

Then, Sarah continued to aid *Reflecting* on the outcome of the visualizing strategies. Through this, Sarah helped Hannah to review what happened as an outcome of implementing their strategies. *(So What?)*

SARAH: Did it *Enable* something new for you? *(So What?)*

HANNAH: I got to know myself better.

1

SARAH: How did it *Feel* to have your *MOW Triangles* in your hands?

HANNAH: It *Felt* really good, because I realized that my life has been *Satisfactory* and I *Feel Happy* with my life so far. And I know better now, where to put my energy more and what needs less effort for now. I have already changed to engage more in our household. My parents noticed it being happy. And my motivation has grown to keep up focused on school.

Now What?

As the process of *Change* on which Hannah and Sarah had agreed seemed to be working well, they continued with their *Plan*.

Sarah's Reflection

Sarah's *Reflection* on their helper-helpee interaction gave her confidence in using the *MOW* and created several questions in her mind about the most accurate and applicable translation of the *MOW* concepts. Drawing on what had happened, Sarah *Reflected* on her own ability as a helper to interact with her helpee as follows:

SARAH: The sessions with Hannah *Felt* like a shared *Doing* for us that we were both keen in learning about and from Hannah to make a *Change* towards what she *Wanted* to achieve. I was genuinely warm, respectful and enthusiastic in working with Hannah. Hannah was my first helpee, and I was eagerly investigating how to apply the *MOW* and communicate it with Hannah the way that assists her in *Feeling Happier* and more *Satisfied* with herself and her life. *(What?)*

Box 9.2 Activities for learning and reflection

Identify someone like a friend or peer who may be interested in the *MOW* and introduce the *MOW* to them. Give yourself 15 minutes for this introduction. Then, using Barton's *3Ws Reflect* on your performance.

What?: What did you choose to focus on from the *MOW*?

So What?: What happened when you explained the *MOW*? Do you think you presented what you wanted to? How did it go? Do you think you will introduce the *MOW* in the same way again?

Now What?: What would you do next time when you want to introduce the *MOW* to someone?

SARAH: It went well and the helper-helpee interaction worked effectively to evaluate Hannah's readiness to continue with the *MOW*. The helper-helpee encounter helped with creating a narrative and coming up with an action plan together to *Empower* Hannah to achieve her *Tailored Triangle*. *(So What?)*

SARAH: The next action for me, however, was to facilitate exploring other *MOW* concepts. *(Now What?)*

Summary

This chapter presented the application of *Reflection* in a *MOW*-based intervention. Examples to illustrate the helper-helpee interaction were presented to aid the helpee's *Reflection*, the helper's *Reflection* and their collaborative *Reflection*.

Further Reading

Barchard, F. (2022). Exploring the role of reflection in nurse education and practice. *Nursing Standard (Royal College of Nursing (Great Britain): 1987)*.

Borton, T. (1970). *Reach, touch and teach*. New York: McGraw-Hill.

Donaghy, M. E., & Morss, K. (2000). Guided reflection: A framework to facilitate and assess reflective practice within the discipline of physiotherapy. *Physiotherapy Theory and Practice*, *16*(1), 3–14.

Gibbs, G. (1988). *Learning by doing: A guide to teaching and learning methods*. London: Further Education Unit.

Grant, A. M. (2022). Reflection, note-taking and coaching: If it ain't written, it ain't coaching!. In D. Tee. & J. Passmore (Eds.), *Coaching Practiced* (pp. 71–83). New Jersey: John Wiley & Sons Ltd.

Li, J. H. (2022). How am I supposed to feel? Female students' emotional reasoning about academic becoming in transnational higher education. *Gender and Education*, 34(5), 560–576.

Ong, M., & Bresman, H. M. (2022). Alone with my thoughts but also my feelings: Neuroticism and the effect of reflection on performance. *Academy of Management Proceedings*. https://journals.aom.org/doi/10.5465/AMBPP.2022.12486abstract

10 Applying the MOW in non-health-related settings

Farzaneh Yazdani and Niayesh Fekri

Box 10.1 Chapter aims

This chapter will cover:

- Examples of employing the *MOW* to investigate a public *Health* issue
- Principles of applying the *MOW* in non–health-related settings
- Health Promotion Models compatible with the *MOW*
- Applying the *MOW* to a work–related problem

This chapter introduces scenarios from different non-health as well as health-related settings in order to demonstrate how the analysis of professional helpees in such situations is conducted and how synthesizing an intervention plan in different contexts can be progressed. The examples covered relate first to the COVID-19 pandemic and then to how help can be extended to individuals or groups seeking help as they are unhappy or dissatisfied with their work or educational aspect of their life. The chapter begins by examining societal influence on *Individuals*.

In spite of individual differences between people, the society they live in has a powerful influence on their mindsets and perspectives. A society influences how people *Think, Feel* and *Do*. On the one hand, this influence is exerted through the laws and regulations enforced by the governing body, and on the other hand, there are culturally held beliefs, taboos and codes of conduct that people may *Feel* they have to adhere to. It is difficult, if not impossible, to truly draw a line that separates an *Individual's* personal beliefs and those held by their family and the wider society or the culture that they live in. People have a tendency to *Do/Not Do* things that ensure social affirmation. As social creatures, the *Need* for survival *Means* that many try to minimize clashes between their personal beliefs and their society. Limiting social circles to people with similar views and perspectives or living within communities that share similar *Values* to those held by an *Individual*, enhances a sense of *Being, Belonging* and *Becoming*. *Self*-Awareness, of an *Individual's Capacities* and *Contextual Factors,* which contributes to what a person can or cannot *Do*, is necessary for their *Well Being* and sense of *Occupational Wholeness (OW)*.

It was explained in Chapter 7 that an *Individual Assigns Meaning* to what they *Do/Not Do*, and the role they consider for themself plays out alongside *Contextual Factors* that influence what they *Do/Not Do* and how they *Do/Not Do*. This chapter explains more

DOI: 10.4324/9781003034759-10

fully how an individual's *Meaning-Making,* which not only infuses what they *Do/Not Do* but also impacts on their *Doings,* is influenced by the society they live in. Accordingly, how the *MOW* can be employed to facilitate the *Well Being* of people in a society is through promoting *Thoughts* that encourage *Realistic* views of people, their *Selves* and their world and their *Choice-Making,* while accepting personal *Responsibility* for their *Choices. Contextual Factors* are strong contributors in forming people's *Triangles* of *Doings.* It was explained earlier that laws and regulations are significant *Contextual Factors* contributing to the way people *Think, Feel* and *Do/Not Do.* Hence, use of the *MOW* is strongly advocated to bring about *Changes* at both individual and public level. In particular, use of the *MOW* should target governing bodies so as to reveal the *Context* that people live in. Several examples are presented in this chapter to demonstrate application of the *MOW* in health and non-health-related public settings.

To present how the *MOW* can be used in a society/community or at general public level, the COVID-19 pandemic 2020 is used as an example of an event that had a noticeable impact on the life and *Well Being* of the public. In exploring people's sense of *Being, Belonging, Becoming* and *OW,* a research project was designed, *the* perceived sense of *Being, Belonging* and *Becoming* during the COVID-19 pandemic measures in mothers of children with disabilities in Iran. This chapter presents selected aspects of what was learned from this project and a proposal for promoting *Change* towards achieving better public *Well Being.*

2020 COVID-19 pandemic

The COVID-19 pandemic was announced by the World Health Organization on March 11, 2020 (https://www.who.int/director-general/speeches/detail/who-director-general-s-opening-remarks-at-the-media-briefing-on-covid-19) with governments across the globe responding in various ways to this declaration. While the issue of the pandemic is a global matter with similarities of impact worldwide, there have been specific consequences of the pandemic and the way it has been managed in each country. The response to the pandemic may be divided into three major paths:

- official rules, regulations and policies announced by governments
- societal and community responses to the pandemic
- societal and community responses to government policies

People's responses in the societies and communities path are the focus of this chapter.

Public interpretation of responses to the COVID-19 pandemic

Evidence shows similarities between contributing factors to stress whether attributed to experience of the COVID-19 pandemic or the ensuing isolation measures. People from lower socio-economic backgrounds faced more severe and often more direct consequences due to the impact of COVID-19 on their everyday life, particularly their employment status, workplace conditions and limitations on accessing support and facilitating services. For instance, the pandemic had a greater negative impact on people with caring responsibilities for children, elderly parents or loved ones with disabilities or long-term conditions. As part of a project studying *Well Being* of the different groups of people in several countries in the Middle East and Europe, in this chapter, the

MOW is used to unfold the stories from women with a caring responsibility as to how sudden *Changes* imposed by the pandemic impacted on this group's sense of *OW*. This group of women was selected due to the complex socio-political status of Iran today and the thought-provoking responses of this group. It is important to be reminded that the COVID-19 pandemic happened in the midst of the United State of America's re-introducing a tighter version of the imposed sanctions on the Islamic Republic of Iran which led to new heights of economic crisis and political turmoil in the country. The extent of economic breakdown in Iran jeopardized the healthcare system and its ability to manage the COVID-19 pandemic.

It is essential for the helpers as individuals or a group of professionals to have a social eye which is sensitive to public issues such as the COVID-19 pandemic. A variety of resources may be used to collect anecdotal evidence based on local knowledge of the situation. To initiate exploration of public issues, anecdotal evidence, such as people's voices on social media platforms for instance, is a valid starting point. For *MOW* professionals, public can mean society at large, particular community groups, or people grouped together based on common characteristics in relation to a phenomenon that they, the helpers, are addressing. For instance, COVID-19 isolation measures had a general impact on the entire society in Iran and globally, but it also had specific impacts on certain groups of people. For instance, healthcare professionals worked during the pandemic everywhere in the world. The impact of the pandemic on healthcare professionals specifically differs from its impact on other groups within a society, such as parents with young children, university students and homeless people. It is meeting the *Needs* of such groups that sometimes interferes with regulatory strategies that address a phenomenon, here, COVID-19, that may concern helpers. The issue of mothers of children with disability was raised by the many Iranian healthcare professionals in the *Context* of working with children with disabilities and their mothers as their main carers. The healthcare professionals acted as the first point of raising an issue about this target group, the mothers of children with a disability, and the need to explore this group and their issues were identified by these healthcare professionals. The next section illustrates an example of an issue that was raised by a group of people, here the mother of children with disabilities as service users of occupational therapy, physiotherapy and speech therapy, that led to a project by a group of Occupational Therapists.

Mothers as carers for children with disabilities in Iran

Hundreds of mothers of children with disabilities who were users of services such as occupational therapy, speech therapy and physiotherapy voiced concerns about limited access to or unavailability of the services during the pandemic in Iran. To understand and respond quickly and effectively to the common issues raised by mothers of children with disabilities, a group of Occupational Therapists from Iran conducted a mixed method (qualitative and quantitative) survey. Several social media groups run by and for mothers of children with disabilities also provided rich data sets to consider. Several Child Occupational Therapists and Speech and Language Pathologists were interviewed by these researchers. To initiate a project to improve the *Well Being* of a public group, this level of information seemed sufficient. In this example, due to the rapid Changes in the situation, quick responses were significant.

Identifying the consensus among the concerns of individuals is highly important when applying the *MOW* at a public level, no matter whether the public group is big or small. The children with disabilities as service users used to spend time outside the home environment while receiving the services available to them. Losing this opportunity impacted on the children's progress in their intervention which caused worries for their mothers in different ways. Some of these worries extended beyond concerns about the interruption to the intervention plan. Scenarios 10.1–10.3, which use pseudonyms, portray examples of some of these concerns that were expressed by mothers of children with disability. These issues could be explained and addressed through a *MOW* filter.

Scenario 10.1

Lili's mother said how difficult it was to explain COVID-19 restrictions to her daughter. She said that she found it difficult to tell Lili the reasons behind her being unable to go outside and meet her grandparents as Lili has a cognitive disability. Lili was often bored at home and her more frequent screaming disturbed her brother's ability to study at home during the period of online schooling.

Scenario 10.2

Giulio's mother said that,

> everyone's at home, my husband is working from home, my other two children are studying from home, and I *Feel* exhausted trying to make peace. Giulio *Needs* a lot of attention, I could let Giulio's little brother play games online at times to keep him busy. But with Giulio it's really hard, due to his physical and visual limitations, to find a substitute for the things he could do in the rehabilitation centre with other children. We just don't have space or equipment. Well, I do find small solutions but I *Feel* exhausted. It's as if I am the centre of keeping everything together. I have no space or time for me.

Scenario 10.3

Mona's therapist mentioned how at first the mothers of the children she had been working with had panicked due to the COVID-19 situation. But after a few sessions of providing her services online, mothers reported interesting *Changes* in their family *Relationships*. She quoted Mona's mother who said, "since my husband is at home and he is not working, he is more involved in implementing Mona's intervention". Mona's mother went on the say that,

> for the first time I *Felt* that my children and my husband are all *Happily* involved in Mona's intervention. We played together and I *Felt* that they appreciated the effort I used to put in to Mona's progress. I *Feel* that we have become closer in understanding each other now that we're working to manage the situation together.

Understanding public narratives is not only about the problems that individuals and groups face but also the ways that different people perceive a problem and their responses to it. Through such understanding, helpers can identify the common problems as well as the potential solutions that people apply leading to their greater *Well Being*.

Understanding public narratives

The three scenarios above (see Scenarios 10.1–10.3) show that while all the mothers of children with a disability *Felt* frustrated due to COVID-19 pandemic restrictions, two mothers experienced only *Negative Thoughts*. In contrast, one mother found *Satisfaction* as an outcome of the COVID-19 restrictions. Readers are reminded that the aim of presenting these examples is not to report the finding of the above research project. These examples are only used to show how issues raised by the mothers of children with disability led to a response from occupational therapists in Iran that potentially could lead to a *MOW*-based project.

Analysing the above examples, the three mothers' worries and *Dissatisfaction* with their respective situation during the COVID-19 pandemic (see Scenarios 10.1–10.3) were reflected in their *Actual Triangles*. The previous *Doings* such as taking their children for their therapy that these mothers were *Valuing* had to stop. Instead, some new *Doings* that were not positively *Meaningful* or *Valued* had to be added to their day-to-day life. *Doings* that these mothers *Felt* was taking away their *Autonomy* and sense of *Control* at times. For two of the mothers, their poorer sense of *Being* was related to an overwhelming sense of *Responsibility* for the *Changes* that needed to be put in place at home, resulting in them having less or no time for themselves to rest or simply *Be* free from *Responsibilities*. The mothers' poorer sense of *Becoming* was related to the ambiguity of the state regarding the pandemic and its impact on their own and their family's future, their loss of hope and their uncertainty about the outcome of the plans they had made. Their poorer sense of *Belonging* related to the authorities' lack of response to the special *Needs* of their children with disability and their own (and/or, their family's) issues. These three mothers were left *Feeling* ignored and left out from the general public. The overall sense of *OW* experienced by these mothers of children with disabilities was that they *Felt* poorer than those whose *Contextual Factors Enabled* them to deal more equitably with the *Unexpected Changes* brought about by the COVID-19 measures. This observation highlights the significance of the need for a project that supports this minority target group at a public level.

In contrast to mothers who showed *Dissatisfaction* with either one or all their *3Bs*, there were also mothers of children with a disability who showed a stronger sense of *Being*, *Belonging*, *Becoming* and an overall greater sense of *OW* during the COVID-19 pandemic measures. These mothers had the following features in common. The presence of partners, other children and grandparents at home who would share *Responsibilities* had an impact on managing the situation. Other family members could take it in turn to implement the intervention for the child with a disability at home. As a result of this collaborative approach at home, mothers could have time to rest or manage working from home with less pressure. In most cases, the sense of *Becoming* and *Belonging* was strongly related to receiving support from their family, as well as from the community, organizations and charities. These positive *Contextual* contributions not only helped to enhance a sense of *Belonging* compared to pre-pandemic times, but also instilled hope for the future. In the case of a stronger sense of *Becoming* amongst the women who were surveyed, there was a distinct link between their *Contextual* support and seeing the future in a more positive way which was something they had not *Expected*.

What has been learnt from the mothers who had a positive experience during the pandemic should be at the core of planning a *MOW*-based project to facilitate a *Tailored Triangle* to strengthen *Being*, *Belonging*, *Becoming* and overall *OW*. A poorer sense of *OW* is not wholly attributable to the limitations of the women's *Actual Triangle* during the pandemic, it is also due to their *Ideal Triangle* which had not been adjusted to the new situation in which the mothers found themself. There is a clear difference between the mothers who had a positive sense of *OW* and *Satisfaction* with their life compared to the group of mothers who had a worse experience during the pandemic and a poorer sense of *OW*. While the former made *Adjustments* to their *Actual Triangles* and had more *Realistic Expectations* about how to manage the pandemic with hope, the latter group had made fewer intentional *Adjustments* to their *Actual Triangles* and *Expectations*. Instead, they had been wishful and had *Expected* the situation to *Change* back to pre-pandemic conditions without taking any steps to *Re-Think* and *Re-Plan* their future. The mothers of children with disabilities who had a positive experience seemed to have made a *Tailored Triangle* in line with the *Changes* that had happened due to the pandemic, whereas the mothers with negative experiences had not made *Change* to their *Expectations* and *Ideals* or their *Actual Doings*.

Overall, while the way that the mothers of children with disabilities responded to the pandemic influenced their *OW*, it was their level of *Contextual* support that played a more significant role in how they managed the COVID-19 pandemic situation. The *Context* was seen to *Empower* and *Enable* mothers in managing their circumstances during the pandemic.

Enhancing the Well Being of the mothers of children with disabilities: a MOW-based project

In identifying the *Need* for helping the mother of children with disabilities as the target group, proposing a *MOW*-based intervention to aid with promoting the *Well Being* of these mothers is established. A deep understanding of narratives, through listening, observing and critical analysis of the mothers' experiences, is essential in *Planning* the *Well Being* project. The aim of the project is to bring about *Change* by developing a *Tailored Triangle* with general principles that facilitated the implementation of the project while allowing the *Autonomy* of the target group. A *Tailored Triangle* needs to be developed to fill the *Gap* between the *Actual* and *Ideal Triangles*. The following section describes the framework of a *Well Being* project for this target group.

Principles of the Well Being Project

The design of the *Well Being Project* targeting the mother of children with disabilities in Iran similar to health promotion projects requires a number of important principles. The success of any *Well Being* project is based on in-depth understanding of the target group and their political and socio–economic *Contexts*. In this section, there is a division between *Change* that focuses on the mothers' role on one hand and their *Context* on the other hand.

A *Tailored Triangle*, consisting of *Enabling* objectives, can be promoted to target both the *Context* and *Empowering* strategies that support individuals and groups. *Empowering* strategies for the individuals in a target group should facilitate the development of problem-solving skills and improve self-efficacy while simultaneously encouraging more *Realistic* beliefs and *Values* about *Change*. The following 12 principles are advised for the above project development.

Principles:

1   In the case of borrowing strategies from other *Contexts* (for instance, other countries, other populations) ensure that the strategies are culturally appropriate to the new *Context* to which it is going to be applied.

2   Use examples of good practice from the cited *Context* above to inform your strategies, for instance, Mothers of children with disabilities with a stronger sense of *Being, Belonging, Becoming* and sense of *OW*.

3   Creative ideas in planning *Well Being* promotion projects need to be sensitive to the cultural, socio-economic and political aspects of the target group's *Context* in order to ensure that their *Tailored Triangle* can be implemented.

4   Educating and training can enhance knowledge and improve the skills needed for *Change*. However, attitudes and beliefs are not easily or quickly *Changeable*.

5   Ensure that the project is suitably flexible to allow *Autonomy* in the *Meaning-Making* of the situation and required *Changes*.

6   *Tailored Triangles* should be explicitly linked to improvement in the overall sense of *OW* and *Self-Fulfilment* to encourage participation.

7   To ensure the success of a *Tailored Triangle*, a step-by-step or graded approach to *Change* is necessary.

8   In situations such as the COVID-19 pandemic, where there is insufficient evidence to support progress, promoting the belief that "every small step is significant" is a key point in *Changing* the *Ideal Triangle*.

9   Allowing a sense of *Autonomy* and *Control* is essential in *Motivating* the target group.

10 Ensure that *Choice-Making* is encouraged and corresponds *Realistically* with the capacities of the *Individuals* and their *Context*.

11 Ensure that a line is drawn between the limitations and restrictions that exist and those perceived by the target group. Aim to decrease limitations and restrictions by practising *Coping* strategies. Working on the person's perception of the situation is key to *Change*.

12 Remember that to improve the overall sense of *OW* and *Well Being*, the project's design should not put *Responsibility* solely on the shoulders of the target group. A *Well Being* project should advocate for the target group in order to secure resources where possible.

Compatibility of the MOW with other models

There are several established health promotion models with which the *MOW* is compatible. Helpers are advised to familiarize themselves with other models when planning their intervention.

This section briefly explains two of the health promotion models that could have been used alongside the *MOW* when planning interventions for the Iranian mothers of children with disabilities.

Health Belief model

The Health Belief (HB) model defines the contributing factors in *Health* behaviours. The key concepts of this model are:

- perceived susceptibility that demonstrates the individual's perceived threat of sickness or disease

- belief of consequence that is related to perceived severity
- potential positive benefits of action
- perceived barriers to action
- exposure to factors that prompt.

According to this model, a person's *Motivation* to undertake a health behaviour intervention depends on individual perceptions, modifying factors and likelihood of action.

The example of the Iranian mothers of children with disabilities during the COVID-19 pandemic is employed here to explain the HB model in the context of the *MOW*. In this *Well Being* project, it was identified that the *Ideal Triangle* of the mothers needed to be *Modified* in accordance with pandemic restrictions. It was shown that while hope was a positive contributing factor for *Changing* in *Doings*, wishful *Thinking* about the situation to resolve itself was a negative contributing factor.

Waiting for the situation to be resolved by itself or by others, *Not Doing* anything to manage the situation and going along with disruption to *Doings* can cost *Individuals* their *Well Being*, *Satisfaction* with themselves and their life. *Thinking* that this situation is not going to impact on their sense of *Being, Belonging, Becoming* and overall *OW* is called perceived susceptibility. While perceived severity refers to lack of acknowledgement about their approach to managing the situation, particularly in the long term, which can create complications.

Not taking action towards *Changing* their *Doings (Actual Triangle)* and their *Expectations* about what is the best thing that can be *Done* in this situation *(Ideal Triangle)* can lead to frustration and *Dissatisfaction*. The overwhelming issue that these mothers had to deal with was their perceived lack of *Control* over *Contextual Factors*, and this barrier prevented them from committing to any *Change* in *Doings*. To develop a *Tailored Triangle*, the *Ideal and Actual Triangles* needed to get closer. In order to facilitate this, the intervention was required to focus on the mothers on the one hand, and their *Context* on the other.

Applying the HB model can help to address the belief-related issues that *Motivated* some mothers and *Demotivated* others, and *Enable* them to participate in a *Well Being* promotion project. The success of the project can be *Predicted* by those target groups that show readiness to *Change* their perspective from wishful *Thinking* to taking action towards developing and implementing the *Tailored Triangle* with hope. As the mothers' belief about their own capacities and abilities to influence their situation was a key factor in adhering to their *Well Being* promotion project, one aspect of the project should therefore focus on improving the mothers' *Self-Awareness* about their own *Capacities*, believing in themselves and using both their personal strengths and their supportive *Contextual Factors*. In the HB model, cues to encourage health behaviours are key elements of health promotion projects. In the *Context* of the Iranian mothers, this concept could have been used to invite and motivate them to *Learn, Practice* and *Reflect* on strategies that could have helped their situation. The *Wholeness Clock* (Figure 10.1) is an example of a prompting device that could have been used through social media as a platform to initiate *Re-thinking* and *Re-planning* and bring about *Change* during the COVID-19 measures.

When planning a *MOW*-based project, social cues can be introduced to help with spreading the Well Being promotion message. An example of such kind of slogan that would attract the attention of the target group, here the mothers of children with disabilities, is shown below.

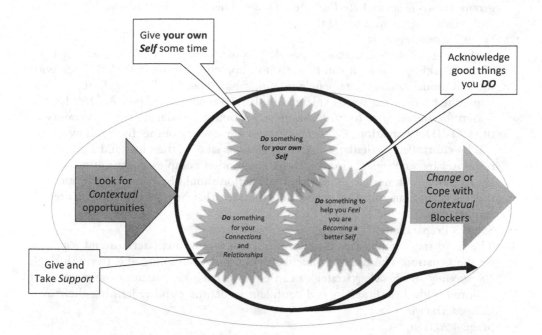

Figure 10.1 The Wholeness Clock

The wholeness clock

The application of ideas for promoting the sense of *OW* at a public level requires precise and clear instructions. The wholeness clock (see Figure 10.1) illustrates an example of a *Self-Tailored* tool to facilitate enhancing *Awareness* about *Doings* to improve *Being, Belonging* and *Becoming*. The wholeness clock offers a simple way towards a *Tailored Triangle* not only for the Iranian mothers of children with disabilities but for all *Individuals* and groups in a *Well Being* project.

The Stage of Behaviour Change model

According to the Stage of Behaviour Change (SoBC) model, the success of *Change* in human behaviour depends on how ready that person is for *Change*, what the barriers they face are and how likely they are to relapse. This model introduces six stages for *Change* as follows:

- Stage 1 Pre-contemplation
  During this stage, people are not considering *Change*. In the example of the mothers of children with disabilities, those mothers with a poorer sense of *OW* who engaged in wishful *Thinking* could be described as 'in denial' according to this model. They did not *Think* that they had to *Change* their *Actual* and *Ideal Triangles* and were waiting for the COVID-19 pandemic situation to return to normal (pre-pandemic situation). Similar to the HB model, at this pre-contemplation stage there is a need for prompting to raise *Awareness* about the necessity of *Individuals* and

groups to *Re-Think* and *Re-Plan* their *Doings*. Therefore, there should be strategies and activities employed to aid this.

- Stage 2 Contemplation
  In this stage of the SoBC model, people become more *Aware* of the potential benefits of making *Change*. It can be seen how applying this model side by side with the HB model can facilitate people moving from Stage 1 to Stage 2. In this second stage, the barriers that were explained in the HB model could be considered as the reason for ambivalence towards taking any action. Considering the uncertainty of the COVID-19 situation, *Changing* views of the severity of the disease, how well it can be controlled particularly with regard to variants of the virus and inconsistent responses by authorities, along with so many other complex contributing factors, led to more confusion about whether any action should be taken. Hence, providing *Contextual* support and advocating the idea that any small action matters is important.

- Stage 3 Preparation
  The third stage emphasizes the significance of taking small actions and *Reflecting* on the situation. The use of problem-solving skills to respond effectively through *Empowering* and *Enabling* strategies can equip participants, such as the mothers of children with disabilities, to *Feel* confident in defining and redefining their own *Tailored Triangle*.

- Stage 4 Action
  This fourth stage is when the *Planned* strategies for *Change* are implemented. In the example of the mothers of children with disabilities, this is when the *Tailored Triangle* of *Doings* is acted upon.

- Stage 5 Maintenance
  Change in *Doings* to which people are habituated is not simple as there is always the temptation to return to old routines. Making a lot of intensive *Changes* in *Doings* within a short period of time requires extensive *Contextual* support in order for participants, such as the mothers, to maintain engagement with the plan. Whilst the mothers' *Self-Awareness* about their abilities and strengths is a significant factor, it is *Unrealistic* and unfair to rely purely on the mothers. The real success of maintaining a target group's engagement with a project to raise their *Satisfaction* with life and *Self-Fulfilment* depends on the contribution of positive *Contextual Factors*. Otherwise, the intervention can turn into another burden for participants, in this case the individual mothers, which contradicts the aim of the intervention. A very important strategy to be used here is the establishment of a reward system to aid with the *Change*.

- Stage 6 Relapse
  Relapse is associated with *Feelings* of frustration, failure and disappointment. In this final stage, helpers should ensure that they have strategies to prevent this from happening by recognizing the barriers and *Reflecting* on the *Tailored Triangle* to ensure that *Change* is within the capacity of the *Individuals* and their *Context*.

The MOW in educational settings during the COVID-19 pandemic

There is a body of knowledge about students' *Satisfaction* with their education. It is natural to think that such a big aspect of students' lives is associated with the overall sense of *OW*: *Satisfaction* with life and *Self-Fulfilment*. Applying the principles of the

MOW within education or work environments may help the *Well Being* of individuals by raising *Self-Awareness* about what contributes to their contentment. The findings of a research project by the author among undergraduate students in Iran and the UK showed that the students encountered disruptions in their *Doings* during the COVID-19 pandemic (Kent & Yazdani, 2020). While the first level of disruption for undergraduate students was related to their education, the *Change* imposed by the COVID-19 measures affected other aspects of their *Doings*, too. The *Changes* in what is *Done* and how it is *Done* resulted in *Changes* in students' sense of *Being, Belonging, Becoming* and *OW*. The closure of the universities and face-to-face education for disciplines such as healthcare education led to missed opportunities for much practical learning that could not be quickly modified for online tutoring. Similar to the findings of the research project related to the mothers of children with disabilities, a division between student experiences was identified. One group formed the majority, within which students presented negative experiences resulting in a poorer sense of *Being, Belonging, Becoming* and *OW*. A smaller group reported positive experiences which provided important knowledge to inform the development of the intervention. The positive experiences came from students who responded to the situation by *Re-thinking, Re-planning* and consequently creating a *Tailored Triangle* in response to the new circumstances. The following characteristics displayed by Zahra, an occupational therapy student, and Marie, an undergraduate student who is married and has a child, were common among this smaller group.

Zahra: I am aware that I'm not able to learn the typical skills that occupational therapy students learn in normal situations but I'm dealing with a real life situation... I have to be creative to modify my services according to the situation we are in now. I'm experimenting with what works online and what doesn't.

Marie: This student reported that during the period of university disruption her husband was at home and receiving benefits from the government. This meant that her husband was able to take more of the childcare responsibilities. Marie herself was able to spend the time that she would have used to commute to the university on attending to tasks she had not been able to before.

Zahra's example shows how she had *Changed* her *Ideal Triangle* by modifying her *Expectations* as well as making the necessary *Changes* to her *Actual Triangle* by performing her practice online. In the second example, the *Contextual* support that Marie received, the financial support from the government and her husband's support with childcare were essential contributing factors, or *Contextual Enablers,* that aid helpees' positive experiences. These kinds of contributing factors should be considered by helpers when planning an intervention project.

Negative student experiences of the COVID-19 impact on universities were mostly associated with the following factors: missing opportunities to connect with other students in person, and lack of support, in particular for those who lived in student accommodation away from their families due to travel restrictions. Students staying at home with their family when their siblings and parents were staying home too found studying difficult. In both situations, whether being alone or being in an overcrowded family home environment had caused difficulties in the *Doing/Not Doing* activities that help form a positive sense of *Belonging*. In turn, such difficulties can affect the sense of *Being*. The sense of *Becoming*, which is related to future prospects, is strongly dependent on *Contextual Factors*. For instance, occupational therapy students in both Iran and the UK did not express any concerns about their future professional life and finding a job. This was because of the way the occupational therapy programmes had responded to the COVID-19 pandemic situation and adjusted the course training, modes and materials. These students also perceived an increase in future demand for their service due to the residual health-related consequences of the COVID-19 pandemic: long-term physical effects of the virus on one hand, and psychosocial and mental *Health* issues on the other hand. However, other healthcare students such as paramedics and physiotherapists showed more worry about their professional future as they *Felt* that the adjustments to their programmes were insufficient for their learning and practice and overall professional competency. Among those students who *Felt* uncomfortable about their learning experiences were a few with a stronger sense of *Becoming*. This group believed that the healthcare system would devise plans, *Contextual support,* to compensate for the learning opportunities they had missed. According to this analysis of the students' circumstances, an intervention that aims to enhance a sense of *Being, Belonging, Becoming* and *OW* should have the following characteristics and be able to:

- Advocate that difficult experiences are opportunities for learning new ways of meeting *Being* needs and connecting and relating to others so as to enhance a sense of *Belonging.*
- Promote learning skills in *Coping* with obligations and build resilience where *Control* over a situation is not possible.
- Acknowledge the limitations and the frustration that come with disruption.
- Engage in *Reflection* to foster knowledge of personal strengths and internalize learning about *Self* as an investment for the future.

The principles that were suggested for planning the intervention for the Iranian mothers of children with a disability apply as equally well in this case of disruption in an education setting. The flexibility of the *MOW* means that it can be used whole or in part for evaluating a public situation or planning a public project. Below is a brief scenario from a *MOW* scholar who has applied the *MOW* in a work environment when the staff *Felt Unhappy* and *Dissatisfied* with their work.

Example of employing the MOW in the workplace

A group of university lecturers working as a team were concerned about the increase in work demands without adequate facilities and support in place. They *Felt* there was no sense of connection among the staff, no sense of "we", and expressed a sense of loneliness.

Many of the members had *Thought* about quitting their job. The helper, a member of the team with the knowledge of the *MOW,* offered to discuss the situation with the team using the *MOW* to explore their issues. She introduced the *Actual* and *Ideal Triangles* to help the team find out about the problem and if they could explain their *Dissatisfaction* through the language of the *MOW* (see Figures 10.2a and 10.2b). The hope was that the *MOW* could assist them in identifying the sources of *Dissatisfaction* and especially the lack of *Belongingness* in the team.

A group discussion showed that the participants *Felt* stressed due to work pressure. Some team members related the pressure to the demands of meeting the required changes in occupational therapy education while there were no changes in salary. They *Felt* that there was not enough support or resources to facilitate responding to the demand of the job. Some team members expressed concern about lack of time and deficiency of

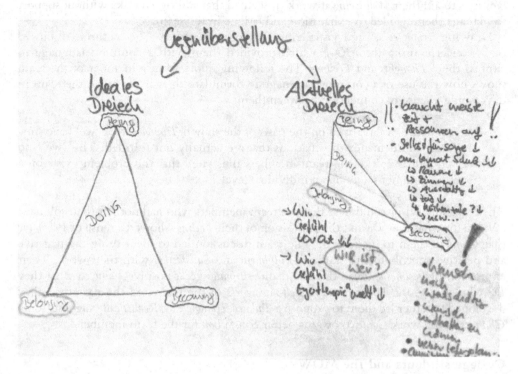

Figure 10.2a The Team Actual Triangle

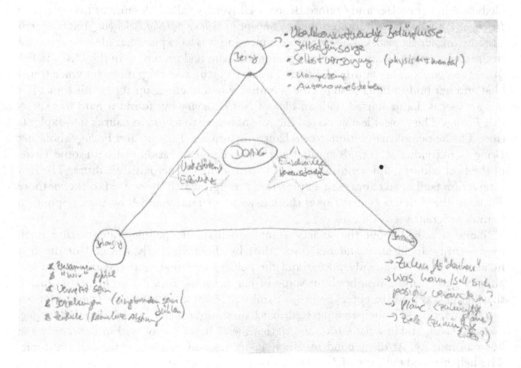

Figure 10.2b The Team Ideal Triangle

facilities to aid their *Well Being* at work. It seemed that additional tasks without support to manage them had led to exhaustion and fatigue in the team.

Drawing *Triangles* assisted visualizing the common issues. The lecturers discussed their concerns using the *MOW* which provided them with a common language to express their *Thoughts* and *Feelings*. The following quote from a member of the team shows how the use of a common language to formulate their issues aided the team in developing a sense of connection between them:

> And suddenly 'we' realized on the basis of the shown *Triangles,* that 'we' have similar *Needs* and demands to situations that are actually not fulfilled. This 'we' and the common *Needs* of the team members illustrated that the problem exists on a structural and not solely on an individual level.

The team supervisor could hear that the team members who had not left their job have a *Value* for what they *Do* and the expression of their *Feelings* showed a sense of *Belonging* that *Connects* them to their work. The team discussion led to identifying the negative and positive contributors to staff *Self-Fulfilment* and *Satisfaction* with their work. Their expression of *Feelings* showed that the team *Attributes* great positive *Value* to what they *Do* wholeheartedly. The collective *Self-Awareness* of the team and the narratives they developed together led them to propose a *Tailored Triangle* that *Realistically* suggests some *Changes* in the work *Context* towards better *Satisfaction* for the team members.

College students and the MOW

Laura, a 19-year-old art student, volunteered for a collaborative project for young people between her college and Oxford Brookes University called "A sense of *Belonging/Not Belonging*". Laura showed interest in the concept of *Belonging/Not Belonging* and used it as a theme for her art pieces. The first project meeting was to explore her ideas and interest in the topic. Laura disclosed how, as a young girl who had grown up in the UK, she *Felt* disconnected from her family and their *Values* as Portuguese migrants. Her voice trembled and her body language showed discomfort when opening up about this topic. For her art pieces, Laura started with an idea of *Not Belonging* but found it hard to express this *Feeling*. The project leader played the role of helper to facilitate Laura's self-exploration. The helper asked questions to aid Laura dig into her *Thoughts* and *Feelings* about her *Being* an individual who finds conflict as a young first-generation girl with some *Values* of the host country, different lifestyle as an art student and her family culture. The first interaction facilitated Laura's self-exploration through which she started to *Become* more *Aware* of the differences she *Thinks* she has with her family and how they respond to Laura's different views on life.

She also talked about the society compartmentalizing people, categorizing them by assigning an identity and her discomfort by these ideas. By the end of the first meeting, Laura was already calmer and the helper's interpretation was that Laura had already gained more insight about some of her *Belonging* issues. The helper evaluated that Laura was ready to enter the project and was given some topics to *Think* of for the second meeting. The helper suggested that Laura might *Think* about partial *Belonging,* *Choice-Making* and in what sense she *Felt* that she *Belonged* or not within her family and her community. At the second meeting, Laura seemed more at ease with the topic. The helper raised the issue of *Meaning-Making* in the context of discovering what Laura

Thinks about integrated *Belonging, Making-Choices* and her likes and dislikes about both her family and community culture. Laura was very receptive to the idea of *Being* able to *Choose* and arriving at an integrated sense of *Belonging*. She was already *Feeling* more positive about her *Choice* of integration rather than dissociation. This *Change* in the way of looking into the topic and bringing *Values* together seemed to have met Laura's sense of *Autonomy* without her needing to fight for her *Choices* and *Feel* uncomfortable about her sense of *Being* either/or.

Throughout the project and discussing ideas about her final piece, Laura went through a journey that enhanced her *Self-Awareness* of what she could *Do/Not Do* in line with what she could *Choose* to *Feel Related* or *Connected* to without *Feeling* being judged, forced or blamed. Laura *Felt* positive about having more *Control* over her sense of *Belonging* and coming up with a solution for integrating what mattered to her from both cultures. She showed more happiness in the way she spoke about her *Feelings* as she *Felt* she was now respectfully *Connected* to both cultural values.

After finalizing her art pieces (see Figures 10.3a and 10.3b), Laura asked her mother and sister to give feedback on their interpretation of her work. It was clear that Laura was excited to share her work with her family and her painting provided a means for her to strengthen her sense of *Belonging* and announce to them how proud she was about it.

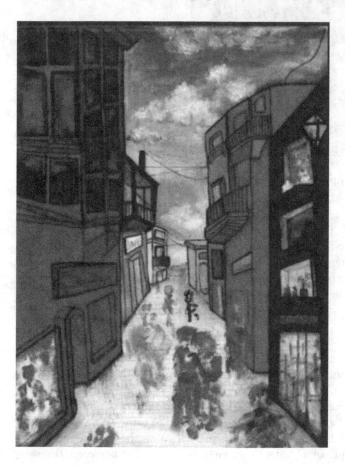

Figure 10.3a Laura's First Art Piece at the Beginning of the Project

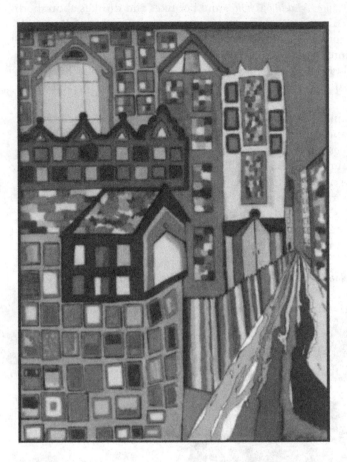

Figure 10.3b Laura's Second Art Piece at the End of the Project

The helper witnessed Laura's *Change* in the way she *Assigned Meaning* to her situation. The significant negative issue in her life at the beginning had *Changed* to become a significant positive *Meaning* where she could see how to be part of both cultures and her *Being* could be a peaceful combination of both. The integration of the sense of *Belonging* led to a sense of integrity in her *Being*.

Summary

The *MOW* was explained using public-level examples from the COVID-19 pandemic. Examples from the mothers of children with a disability and healthcare students were used to demonstrate how the *MOW* can be implemented at community/social level. To show an application of the *MOW* in a workplace environment, another example addressed a conflict that had resulted in staff *Dissatisfaction* and low sense of *Belonging* among a group of professionals. An application of the *MOW* in the context of college students presented an example of a student's journey from conflict between *Belonging* and *Not Belonging* through to developing a narrative of integration presented in art pieces.

Box 10.2 Activities for learning and reflection

With your peers discuss

1 Anecdotal evidence that might be investigated through the *MOW.*
2 A target group with a common issue that may be addressed through the *MOW.*

Further reading

Asa, G. A., Fauk, N. K., Ward, P. R., Hawke, K., Crutzen, R., & Mwanri, L. (2021). Psychological, sociocultural and economic coping strategies of mothers or female caregivers of children with a disability in Belu district, Indonesia. *PLoS One, 16*(5), e0251274.

Cacioppo M, Bouvier S, Bailly R, Houx L, Lempereur M, Mensah-Gourmel J, Kandalaft C, Varengue R, Chatelin A, Vagnoni J, Vuillerot C, Gautheron V, Dinomais M, Dheilly E, Brochard S, Pons C; ECHO Group. (2021). Emerging health challenges for children with physical disabilities and their parents during the COVID-19 pandemic: The ECHO French survey. *Annals of Physical and Rehabilitation Medicine, 64*(3), 101429.

Castro-Kemp, S., & Mahmud, A. (2021, May). School closures and returning to SCHOOL: Views of parents of children with disabilities in England during the Covid-19 pandemic. *Frontiers in Education6*, 666574. doi: 10.3389/feduc.2021.666574

Cerulo, K. A., Leschziner, V., & Shepherd, H. (2021). Rethinking culture and cognition. *Annual Review of Sociology, 47*, 63–85.

Davis, A. S., Kafka, A. M., González-Morales, M. G., & Feitosa, J. "(2022). Team belonging: Integrating teamwork and diversity training through emotions. *Small Group Research, 53*(1), 88–127.

Farajzadeh, A., Dehghanizadeh, M., Maroufizadeh, S., Amini, M., & Shamili, A. (2021). Predictors of mental health among parents of children with cerebral palsy during the COVID-19 pandemic in Iran: A web-based cross-sectional study. *Research in Developmental Disabilities, 112*, 103890.

Godor, B. P., & Van der Hallen, R. (2022). Investigating the susceptibility to change of coping and resiliency during COVID-19. *Scandinavian Journal of Psychology, 63*(3), 238–245.

Gopalan, M., Linden-Carmichael, A., & Lanza, S. (2022). College students' sense of belonging and mental health amidst the COVID-19 pandemic. *Journal of Adolescent Health, 70*(2), 228–233.

Green, J., Cross, R., Woodall, J., & Tones, K. (2019). *Health promotion: Planning and strategies* (4th ed.). Sage.

Hauf, P., & Friedrich, F. (2007). *Making minds: The shaping of human minds through social context* (Ser. Benjamins current topics, v. 4). John Benjamins Pub. Retrieved July 22, 2022, from: https://ebin.pub/making-minds-the-shaping-of-human-minds-through-social-context-benjamins-current-topics-9027222347-9789027222343-9789027292742.html

Kavanagh, S., Shiell, A., Hawe, P., & Garvey, K. (2022). Resources, relationships, and systems thinking should inform the way community health promotion is funded. *Critical Public Health, 32*(3), 273–282.

Kent, J. Yazdani, F. (2020). *Impact of COVID-19 on student and newly qualified healthcare professionals: A qualitative approach.* Unpublished MSc Dissertation. Oxford Brookes University.

Lades, L. K., Laffan, K., Daly, M., & Delaney, L. (2020). Daily emotional well-being during the COVID-19 pandemic. *British Journal of Health Psychology, 25*(4), 902–911.

Leitch, S., Corbin, J. H., Boston-Fisher, N., Ayele, C., Delobelle, P., Gwanzura Ottemöller, F., Matenga, T. F. L., Mweemba, O., Pederson, A., & Wicker, J. (2021). Black lives matter in health promotion: Moving from unspoken to outspoken. *Health Promotion International, 36*(4), 1160–1169.

Prime, H., Wade, M., & Browne, D. T. (2020). Risk and resilience in family well-being during the COVID-19 pandemic. *American Psychologist*, 75(5), 631.

Ramaswamy, M., & Freudenberg, N. (2022). Health promotion in jails and prisons: An alternative paradigm for correctional health services. In R.B. Greifinger, (Eds.), *Public health behind bars* (pp. 219–238). New York: Springer.

Szelei, N., Devlieger, I., Verelst, A., Spaas, C., Jervelund, S. S., Primdahl, N. L., Skovdal, M., Opaas, M., Durbeej, N., Osman, F., Soye, E., Colpin, H., De Haene, L., Aalto, S., Kankaanpää, R., Peltonen, K., Andersen, A. J., Hilden, P. K., Watters, C., & Derluyn, I. (2022). Migrant students' sense of belonging and the Covid-19 pandemic: Implications for educational inclusion. *Social Inclusion*, 10(2), 172–184.

Walters, T., & Venkatachalam, T. S. (2022). The difference Diwali makes: Understanding the contribution of a cultural event to subjective well-being for ethnic minority communities. *Event Management*, 26(1), 141–155.

Walther, C. C. (2022). Compassion for change. Nurturing the motivation of Staff in UN institutions dedicated to the promotion of human rights. *The International Journal of Human Rights*, 26(8), 1455–1475

Wang, L. (2022). Belonging, being and becoming: Tertiary students in China in the battle against COVID-19 pandemic. *STAR Scholar Book Series*, 39–56.

Yazdani, F., Nazi, S., Kavousipor, S., Karamali Esmaili, S., Rezaee, M., & Rassafiani, M. (2021). Does covid-19 pandemic tell us something about time and space to meet our being, belonging and becoming needs? *Scandinavian Journal of Occupational Therapy*, 1–10. https://www.tandfonline.com/doi/full/10.1080/11038128.2021.1994644, accessed July 2022.

Yazdani, F., Rezaee, M., Rassafiani, M., Roberts, D., Abu-Zurayk, W., & Amarlooee, M. (2021). The COVID-19 pandemic may force the world to reflect on the pre-pandemic style of life. *International Journal of Travel Medicine and Global Health*, 9(3), 124–131.

11 Applying the MOW in in-patient and out-patient settings

Farzaneh Yazdani

Box 11.1 Chapter aims

This chapter will cover:

- The application of a *MOW*-based intervention in in-patient and out-patient hospital settings
- A protocol to facilitate a *MOW*-based intervention with patients
- Two scenarios to demonstrate a *MOW*-based intervention at different levels of patient readiness

---

This chapter explores a *MOW*-based intervention with a group of people commonly considered as patients who seek occupational therapy services related to their ill health. Their therapy can take place within a hospital environment, as with other in-patients and out-patients, or through follow-up services in community settings. The chapter demonstrates how analysis of a helpee's situation and the design of their intervention plan can proceed.

All hospital settings are subject to restrictions informed by health policies and regulations. These protocols dictate the time and duration of the interventions that are in place for different patients. The services provided along with the job description of healthcare professionals working at hospitals are widely regulated by the health system in each country.

With regard to the *MOW,* a helper can be any healthcare professional who, within the capacity of their job description, is able to apply any aspect of the model in their practice. There are essential factors to consider when applying the *MOW* with *Individuals*. First, a helper with knowledge of the philosophy and principles of the *MOW* can use their professional reasoning to completely or partially implement the *MOW*. In either case, the helper's professional reasoning guides them to identify which aspects of the *MOW* are likely to be usefully addressed within the time frame of the hospitalization or discharge plan and the *Needs* of the patients. The issue of partial application of the *MOW* is not restricted to interventions with individuals or hospital settings. The significance of applying the *MOW* is in understanding and conceptualizing the philosophy and principles of the model, integrating that with other compatible models (see Chapter 10) and using professional reasoning as to when and how to use the *MOW* to aid helpees. The phases and steps of a *MOW*-based intervention as discussed in chapter 6

DOI: 10.4324/9781003034759-11

show how helpers can employ a systematic process of professional reasoning that may be simplified depending on the circumstance. In the following section, the examples presented demonstrate simplified applications of the *MOW* in three different circumstances. When reading the examples, it should be borne in mind that hospitals in different countries have different protocols for interventions, from referral to discharge. The next section begins with a protocol for a *MOW* intervention plan.

Intervention protocol: the rule of 'SEVEN'

- **Step1 Understanding people and their narratives (**Identifying the problem)
  Based on the *MOW,* the identified problem is that the person is not *Satisfied* with themselves or their life situation. To use *MOW* terminology, the person is *Unhappy* or *Dissatisfied* with either one, two or all of their *3Bs of Being, Belonging and Becoming* or their *Doings.* Therefore, when the person is seen by a helper, whether therapist or healthcare professional, they should assess whether this person's problem makes them eligible for a *MOW*-based intervention. The following issues are among those that may be addressed through the *MOW* in in-patient or out-patient settings:
  1   Overall negative *Feeling* about *Self* and life due to ill health
  2   *Dissatisfaction* with their *Being, Belonging* and *Becoming* and how to meet these *Needs* given their ill health
  3   Problem with identifying the link between *Doings* and meeting the *Needs* of *Being, Belonging* and *Becoming* due to the influence of ill health
  4   Problem with formulating *Change* even when the person has realized it is required
  5   Problem in identifying *Contextual Factors* and their role in *Doings*
  6   Confusion or lack of insight into how significant *Meanings* of their situation impacts on them negatively and positively
  7   Problem in linking the *Choice-Making, Assigning Meaning* and *Attribution* of *Values* to *Doings* and events and the way these influence their *Well Being*
  People who are keen to consider *Re-thinking* and *Re-planning* their life would also be eligible to receive a *MOW* intervention. Eligibility, therefore, is indicated when a person is interested in raising *Self-Awareness* about the state of their own *OW* comprising their *Doings* and sense of *Being, Belonging* and *Becoming.* These people may be included in a *MOW*-based intervention based on their interests in *Reflecting* on their world/life, *Doings* and *Thinking* patterns and *Re-thinking* and *Re-planning* their life.
- **Step 2 Identifying the Disharmony and Incongruence/Gap**
  In this second step, the helper and helpee should deepen their understanding of the links between the helpee's *Doings* and the ways they meet, or do not meet, their *Being, Belonging* and *Becoming Needs.* To achieve this aim, the helper needs to explain the *MOW* concepts in language that can be understood readily by the helpee (see Table 11.1). Communicating the basic principles of the *MOW* is vital for the helpee's understanding and outcome of the intervention. The concepts below are arranged in the order in which they might be introduced in an intervention.
- **Step 3 Conceptualizing the Change that needs to be made**
  To establish strategies for *Change,* helpers and helpee need to:
  1   Determine limitations and restrictions that have caused the gap from an *Individual* and *Contextual* perspective.

Table 11.1 The MOW Concepts in Lay Language

MOW theoretical concept	MOW concept in lay language
Occupational Wholeness	This is your perception of life situations when you are *Satisfied* with your life and *Feel/Think* relatively well about it.
Doings	Your actions, what you *Do* or intentionally *Not Do*.
Being	The way you see yourself, what you like, the way to be genuinely *Happy* or *Satisfied*, and gives you a sense of joy or comfort, *Feeling* of *Control* over your own life.
Belonging	Who you like to be with, spend time with and share space with. Place you *Value* or enjoy being, where you like to visit and *Feel* at home. Ideas you *Think* define your *Values*, and the people/places, and ideas you *Feel* part of.
Becoming	Your future plan, what you hope for, where you want to be in the future and who you would like to *Become*.
Actual Triangle	What you *Do/Not Do* in your life to aid *Feeling* good about yourself, your life and your future plans. What you *Do/Not Do* that aids your being with people you like and *Connect* with. What makes you *Feel* related to people, places and ideas that make you *Happy* or *Satisfied* with your life and help you *Feel* content.
Ideal Triangle	What you wish/prefer/*Value Doing/Not Doing* that you believe makes you *Feel* good about yourself. Your future plans and people/places/ideas you *Feel* part of.
Tailored Triangle/Reality Triangle	*Doings* and/or *Thoughts* that are realistic and achievable within an agreed period of time to aid your *Satisfaction* and *Happiness*.
Congruence/ Incongruence	When the state of your current life situation and what you *Value*, prefer or wish for, almost point in one direction, there is a *Congruence*. When they fall apart and take different directions, there is an *Incongruence* between your acts and *Needs*.
Harmony/Disharmony	If what you *Do/Not Do* to meet one *Need* aids others, it is called *Harmony*. But when acting to meet one of your *Needs* makes you distant from the other, or even goes against meeting the other *Need*, it is called *Disharmony*.
Skewed Triangle	When what you *Do/Not Do Satisfies* one or two of your *Needs* in an exaggerated manner that denies the others, it is called a skew. A skewed *Triangle* is recognized by its uneven/irregular shape.
Contextual Factors (positive)	Elements around you that help you to *Do/Not Do* things that are in your favour.
Contextual Factors(negative)	Elements around you that do not help you and may even work against your *Doing/Not Doing* things that are in your favour.
Changeability	When factors that you *Think* contribute to your life are considered to have the potential for *Change* and are not fixed.
Coping	When you face *Unchangeable* situations and you need to accept and find a way to deal with them as they are.
Obligation	Elements of your *Context* that are either *Unchangeable* or only *Changeable* if much investment is required to the extent that you find it impossible or extremely difficult to make it happen.
Choice-Making	A decision-making process that starts with identifying the options that are available to *Choose* from.
Assignment of *Meaning* or *Meaning-Making* (negative or positive)	The way you explain an event, act or situation that provokes a positive or negative *Feeling* in you.
Attributing Value	How you evaluate an event, act or situation and its worth from your own point of view.

2   Identify available facilitators and opportunities which indicate what, potentially, can and cannot *Change*.

3   Identify which aspect of *Change* is more significant (positively *Meaningful*) for the person and how much *Change* is *Satisfactory*.

4   Ask/ascertain/clarify/agree what *Changes* need to be made in *Actual Doings* given the person's *Contextual* opportunities and *Individual* capacities.

5   Ask/ascertain/clarify/agree what *Changes* need to be made in the *Ideal Triangle* to bring it closer to *Reality*.

6   Develop a *Reality*-based *Triangle/Tailored Triangle* which is a compromise between the person's *Actual* and *Ideal Triangles* underpinned by positive *Meanings* and *Values*.

7   Agree when and where to start the intervention/the process of *Change*.

- **Step 4 Identifying the person's Readiness for Change**
  The intervention plan differs depending on the person's *Readiness* for initiating the process of *Change*. If the helpee is not *Ready* to be entered in a *MOW*-based intervention, the helper needs to decide whether they have the potential to be *Prepared* for a *MOW*-based intervention and accordingly apply strategies to *Prepare* them.

  1   What is the helpee's belief about people's capacity for *Change* in general?

  2   What is their belief about the role of a person's *Context* in general?

  3   What do they *Think* about their own ability to *Change*?

  4   What do they *Think* about the level of *Control* they may have over their own *Doings and Thinking* or their own *Context*?

  5   Do they show interest in general/in the *MOW*?

  6   Do they *Value Change*?

  7   Can you, as the helper, identify at which stage of *Change* they are? See Chapter 10 for the Stage of Behaviour Change (SoBC) model: pre-contemplation, contemplation, commitment, action, sustained or leave.

- **Step 5 Planning the strategies**
  The helper and helpee create the *Tailored Triangle*. *Meaning-Making, Choice-Making* and *Responsibility* for *Change* are used as fundamental *MOW* principles to establish the *Tailored Triangle*. Following analysis of the stage the person is at, regarding their commitment to *Change* and collaboration on the *Plan* to *Change*, the following strategies are introduced to *Enable* and *Empower* the *Individual* to *Change*. Strategies to facilitate *Change*:

  1   Using problem-solving approaches.

  2   Adapting/Modifying *Thinking* processes to aid the helpee's evaluation of *Reality*.

  3   Ensuring sustainability of the *Change*.

  4   Modifying the helpee's *Contexts*.

  5   *Planning* pragmatically.

  6   Acknowledging and *Valuing Change*.

  7   Enjoying the *Change*.

- **Step 6 Implementing the strategies**
  The *MOW*-based intervention plan emphasizes practice-based learning in all areas of *Thinking, Feeling* and *Doing*. From the following list, helpers need to make a

decision as to which method of intervention would be more beneficial and practically available for the helpee:

1 Method of delivery: individual, group or both.
2 Exercises and activities.
3 Effective schedule for planning practice.
4 Reinforcing factors? Methods/tools– for practice.
5 Record-keeping system for practice.
6 Key factors facilitating sustainability.
7 Indicators of the areas for re-evaluation.

• **Step 7 A final summative Reflection**
The helper and helpee need to *Reflect* on the *Changes* they *Thought* of, *Planned* for and implemented. This can be done together and/or separately. The final summative *Reflection* can address the intervention plan in part or in its entirety. The helper and helpee *Reflection* steps follow:

1 Decide on the part of the intervention they *Need*/wish to *Reflect* on.
2 Choose a *Reflection* model from Chapter 9
3 Agree whether the helper and helpee need to *Reflect* separately or together.
4 Decide how to implement the *Reflection*: writing, audiovisual recording, drawing, etc.
5 Implement the *Reflective* exercise.
6 Meet to discuss their respective *Reflections*.
7 Decide whether the action plan includes discharging the helpee from the *MOW* or continuing.

Examples of applying the *MOW* in a hospital setting using the *MOW* protocol are presented in Scenarios 1 and 2 below.

Scenario 1

Althea, Mila's mother, had a transient ischemic attack (TIA) during pregnancy. This mini-stroke left her with mild- to moderate-level apraxia which affects her speech. Her baby, Mila, was born prematurely with some complications to her lung and heart functions. She needed to stay in the hospital until her situation improved. Mila is Althea's first child. Althea is 22 years old and her partner is 28, both work full time. The medical team at the hospital has planned for Mila's parents to visit Mila and stay with her to help with Mila's transition from the hospital to home. A healthcare support plan for Mila has been put in place by the hospital. Mila's father, though, is extremely anxious as he finds it difficult to manage the demands of his job and the new family circumstances. The maternity leave for Althea permits a maximum of eight weeks. However, there are no such contractual rights to paternity leave in the country where they live. The focus of this scenario is on the situation from Althea's perspective.

Althea feels confused about the entire situation, saying,

> I was about to submit my promotion application which would have helped me financially when my baby arrives. My TIA and Mila's premature birth changed everything. It just feels like there is a lot to deal with right now. I have to get on with the healthcare plan I have been given for myself…(cries)…Mila is ill and I can't even hold her.

Step1 Understanding people and their narratives

Althea's life situation has undergone huge *Change*, especially her sense of *Being* as a new mother to Mila. The process of preparation for her role as a mother was disrupted by the premature birth of her child and the complications that have arisen from it. Her *Plans* for promotion that were aligned with her preparations for *Becoming* a mother have been upset. The process of bonding with her child through physical touch and breastfeeding has not begun as her daughter is in hospital. Due to Althea's inability to execute her *Plans,* she *Feels* frustrated about her (perceived) lack of *Doings.* She seems to be *Dissatisfied* with her lack of *Control* over the situation. The helper's professional evaluation is that Althea is eligible to be entered into a *MOW*-based intervention plan. The helper decides to aid Althea in reviewing her options through evaluating her personal and *Contextual* capacities. The helper, therefore, discusses with Althea the idea of drawing her *Actual* and *Idea Triangles* and subsequently her *Tailored Triangle* over a period of one month, which is the duration of Mila's stay in the hospital and the length of Althea's healthcare support. This scenario is informed by a real situation. A *MOW*-based terminology is used to analyse this scenario. Pseudonyms have been used.

Step 2 Identifying the Disharmony, Discrepancy/Gap

It is clear that Althea's *Actual Triangle* is small and tending towards negative scores that demonstrate how she has evaluated her *Actual Doings* towards meeting her *3B Needs* negatively (see Figure 11.1). There is *Disharmony* between her *Becoming* and *Belonging Needs* in particular and the overall the *Discrepancy/Gap* is huge.

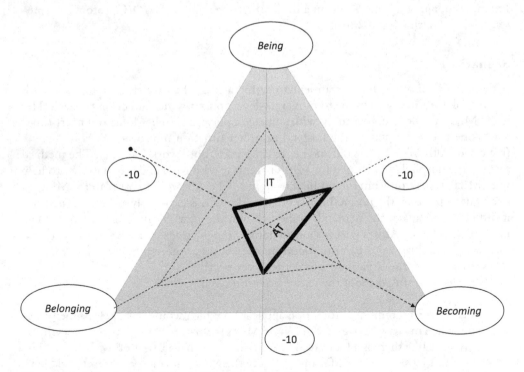

Figure 11.1 Althea's *Actual Triangle*, Disharmony and Incongruence

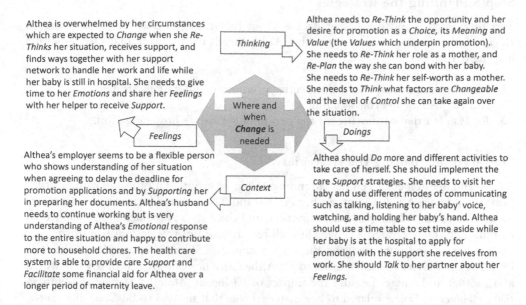

Althea is overwhelmed by her circumstances which are expected to *Change* when she *Re-Thinks* her situation, receives support, and finds ways together with her support network to handle her work and life while her baby is still in hospital. She needs to give time to her *Emotions* and share her *Feelings* with her helper to receive *Support*.

Thinking

Althea needs to *Re-Think* the opportunity and her desire for promotion as a *Choice*, its *Meaning* and *Value* (the *Values* which underpin promotion). She needs to *Re-Think* her role as a mother, and *Re-Plan* the way she can bond with her baby. She needs to *Re-Think* her self-worth as a mother. She needs to *Think* what factors are *Changeable* and the level of *Control* she can take again over the situation.

Feelings

Where and when *Change* is needed

Doings

Althea's employer seems to be a flexible person who shows understanding of her situation when agreeing to delay the deadline for promotion applications and by *Supporting* her in preparing her documents. Althea's husband needs to continue working but is very understanding of Althea's *Emotional* response to the entire situation and happy to contribute more to household chores. The health care system is able to provide care *Support* and *Facilitate* some financial aid for Althea over a longer period of maternity leave.

Context

Althea should *Do* more and different activities to take care of herself. She should implement the care *Support* strategies. She needs to visit her baby and use different modes of communicating such as talking, listening to her baby' voice, watching, and holding her baby's hand. Althea should use a time table to set time aside while her baby is at the hospital to apply for promotion with the support she receives from work. She should *Talk* to her partner about her *Feelings*.

Figure 11.2 Analysis of the Need for Change for Althea

Step 3 Conceptualizing the Change that needs to be made

Althea, understandably upset over Mila's lengthy stay in hospital as well as her own physical and mental issues, *Feels* overwhelmed by the entire situation. Naturally, it takes time before she can manage her emotions and be able to *Re-Think* and *Re-Plan* her life situation. As part of her intervention, the helper needs to facilitate the *Context* so as to permit Althea to express her *Feelings*. The helper needs to use empathetic listening skills to aid this. When Althea *Feels* more *Control* over her emotions, together with the helper they can start *Re-thinking* the entire situation and *Re-planning* for the period of time while the baby is in hospital. Figure 11.2 illustrates what may or may not need *Changing* to help Althea during this period.

Step 4 Identifying the person's Readiness for Change

Althea is happy to start being able to see the whole situation through the lens of the *MOW*. She is eager to help herself and improve her family life and said, "The *MOW* philosophy sounds interesting, I would like to try it as I really want to take control over my life again and I am confident that I will if I just learn how". Althea's insight about her ability to *Control* some aspects of her situation and her *Motivation* towards initiating this process using the *MOW* shows her readiness for *Change*. Her *Context* is supportive and some facilities are already available to her. Additionally, the helper's evaluation of Althea's situation is positive, and the helper suggests that they start their sessions as soon as possible.

Step 5 Planning the strategies

Together, Althea and her helper decide about the strategies that would help her to *Re-Think* the situation. They agree that Althea needs to use three main strategies for helping her to:

1 Explore the *Meaning* of the prospective promotion and its *Value* to her
2 Aid *Re-thinking* her role as a mother
3 *Re-Plan* her day-to-day life for the period of her baby's hospitalization.

Step 6 Implementing the strategies

Althea and her helper agreed that attending a support group of mothers in similar situations would help Althea to express her *Feelings* and *Thoughts* and hear others' comments in relation to the *Meaning* of her promotion, and the *Values Attributed* to her self-worth as a mother. They created a timetable with rewards for positive actions towards taking care of herself and implementing the agreed strategies. The helper employed the Balloon Person activity (see Chapter 8) to aid Althea's *Re-thinking* process of her self-worth as a mother and gauge/measure the impact of *Change* in *Meaning-Making* and *Attribution* of *Values* to *Doings* related to her maternal role that needed to be *Done* differently. Through this Balloon Person activity, the helper aimed to *Empower* Althea to *Make Choices* and enhance her *Self-Awareness* about the impact of her *Choices* on her sense of *Being, Belonging* and *Becoming*. Althea and her helper also used collage making to aid Althea's expression of her interests and *Values* in *Doings* that facilitated her *Being Need* in particular.

Step 7 A final summative Reflection

In this out-patient *MOW*-based intervention, the helper assisted Althea in drawing up a personalized plan that facilitated Althea's process of *Reflection* that lead to an action plan in preparation for the discharge of her hospitalized baby.

Scenario 2

The second scenario shows how a helper's professional reasoning supported a *MOW*-based intervention with a hospitalized patient initially reluctant to participate. The scenario is informed by a real story in which a pseudonym is used. Matine, the in-patient in this scenario, faces *Changes* in his life due to a health condition that impacts on his *Doings*. The scenario shows how Matine's sense of *Being, Belonging* and *Becoming* is affected by his illness.

Matine, 60 years old, is hospitalized due to myocardial infarction (MI). He is a secondary school teacher who has undergone open-heart surgery, and his recovery plan includes sick leave for three months and several restrictions on his *Doings*. He used to walk the 25-minute distance between his house and school everyday. Matine also used to shop for groceries on his way back and cook after work for himself and his wife who is a teacher, too. Their two children have grown up and live in other cities, one and three hours' driving distance away, respectively. Matine enjoyed cooking, long walks at weekends and visiting his children and grandchildren. Following surgery, Matine is not allowed to walk long distances for the first month after his discharge. He finds the recovery plan very restrictive, does not believe in taking rest and resists staying at home. His wife and children are worried that he will become depressed if forced to be less active than before. Matine's wife is anxious that she may not be able to manage the situation on her own. Matine says, with an expression of despair, "She cannot manage without me *Doing* the shopping and cooking and no way will I stay home. We *Need* food and I won't allow my heart issues to turn me into a useless *Being*". His frustration and unhappiness are increased when told that he cannot return to work immediately. Matine's sense of *Belonging* to his school and his self-worth that he associates with his role as a teacher and supportive husband are shaken. He is worried that because of his heart attack, he may be forced into early retirement which goes against his previous plan of *Becoming* the school principal before retirement.

The hospital care team is in agreement that as Matine's health and consequently his life situation have *Changed*, they need to aid him in *Re-thinking* and *Re-planning* his future life. Matine's social worker is a *MOW*-trained professional who offers to act as his helper to aid the team with implementing a care plan. Matine seems to be not *Ready* for entering a *MOW*-based intervention so the helper needs to *Prepare* him for that first. The helper invites Matine's wife and their two children to meet up and discuss the situation. The helper hopes that the meeting with the family may help to prepare Matine for a *MOW*-based intervention.

According to the Stage of Behaviour Change model (see Chapter 10), Matine is at a pre-contemplation stage. Therefore, the helper needs to use strategies to *Motivate* Matine to move to the next step. In Chapter 10, two health promotion models were briefly introduced. Although these models were originally developed to be used at a public level, the principles and strategies of both models can be applied at an individual level. In Chapter 6, the decision–making diagram (see Figure 6.1) showed that helpers need to prepare potential helpees if their professional reasoning suggests that they might usefully benefit from a *MOW*-based intervention but not *Ready* to be entered into it straight away. The helper, therefore, needs to apply strategies to *Prepare* the person. In Matine's case, the helper evaluates Matine's situation also from the perspective of the Health Belief model (see Chapter 10). It appears that Matine does not evaluate his heart condition as being as severe as his medical team believes. He also thinks the consequences of not committing himself to the care plan to be unharmful. The helper, however, understands that Matine is a confident person who believes in his abilities to *Control* his life situation in general. The helper's evaluation of the situation is that Matine lacks knowledge of his condition and underestimates his wife's ability to manage the situation alone. Although Matine's wife expressed concern and showed low confidence in managing their life without Matine's help/input, the helper's evaluation of her capacities is that she would be able to take more *Responsibilities* if needed and is only worried as she is not used to it. In other words, while the sudden *Changes* in their life pattern have caused them both concern, they need to face their new *Reality* which they should be able to *Cope* with provided they are educated and given enough time to *Think* about the situation differently. The helper believes that Matine and his wife need to *Re-Think* and *Re-Plan* their *Doings*. The helper's meeting with the family is to identify how much support Matine and his wife can expect to receive from their children, if required, and to confront them all with the new situation that needs to be reviewed. The helper hopes to encourage Matine to *Reflect* on his strengths in dealing with the *Changes* required, educate all family members about the severity of Matine's condition and the significance of making *Choices* that can help with his life in the long term. The helper's *Plan* is to then move to the next step which is entering Matine and his wife into a *MOW*-based intervention.

The helper needs to use encouraging strategies to *Empower* Matine to *Reflect* on his abilities in managing his situation. As Matine is a teacher, the helper hypothesizes that Matine may *Change* towards more collaboration with the helper and the care team if he is educated more about his condition. The helper, therefore, provides Matine with pamphlets and educational videos hoping that these may *Change* his attitude towards his care plan, show his susceptibility to a worsened heart condition and how beneficial it would be to commit himself to the care plan. Through this strategy, the helper predicts that Matine may move to a contemplation stage and be *Readier* to start the *MOW*-based intervention. The helper relies on Matine's family to show their support.

At the subsequent meeting with Matine and his family, the helper began by validating Matine's *Feelings* and acknowledged that this sudden *Change* in his work and family life must have been a shock to him. Matine then declared his frustration about how his life plans are obstructed by his MI and long hospitalization. The helper asked Matine about his understanding of his condition and realized that he had not been fully informed that his surgical procedure is classified as a major heart operation that requires a post-operative intervention to ensure success of the treatment. The helper educated Matine and his family about the necessity of committing to the care plan after his discharge. Matine listened carefully and seemed to realize the severity of his condition and the *Value* of the postoperative intervention *Plan*. While his body language conveyed his disappointment, Matine mentioned his concern about his routines and how everything would be upside down. He showed worry for his wife and students and expressed concern that he may not be able to manage everything. The helper introduced the idea of a *MOW*-based intervention to support him and his family to formulate a *Plan* to aid them all to work together and towards managing the situation. The helper's brief about the way the *MOW* could be of help interested Matine and his family who decided to participate. Matine himself, in particular, showed more motivation and some knowledge of a *MOW*-based interventions. All family members agreed to attend a second group meeting to aid the helper and Matine agree a *Tailored Triangle* that includes identifying roles for Matine's wife and children, too.

Summary

This chapter presented two scenarios to show how a *MOW*-based intervention can be used alongside other interventions in a hospital to aid patients' *Re-thinking* and *Re-planning* their life situation under different health circumstances. The first scenario looked at issues encountered by a mother after giving birth to a baby with health conditions. The second scenario explored the *Readiness* and the process of entering a patient and his family into a *MOW*-based intervention concurrent with postoperative treatment and a discharge care plan.

Box 11.2 Activities for learning and reflection

Read Matine's scenario again carefully and draw his *Actual* and *Ideal Triangles* and then suggest a *Tailored Triangle* assuming that Matine accepts support from his wife and children.

Further Reading

Alizadeh, S., Khanahmadi, S., Vedadhir, A., & Barjasteh, S. (2018). The relationship between resilience with self-compassion, social support and sense of belonging in women with breast cancer. *Asian Pacific Journal of Cancer Prevention: APJCP, 19*(9), 2469.

Callanan, J., Signal, T., & McAdie, T. (2021). What is my child telling me? Reducing stress, increasing competence and improving psychological well-being in parents of children with a developmental disability. *Research in Developmental Disabilities, 114*, 103984.

Cappo, D., Mutamba, B., & Verity, F. (2021, March 12). Belonging home: Capabilities, belonging and mental health recovery in low resourced settings. *Health Promotion International 36*(1), 58–66. https://doi.org/10.1093/heapro/daaa006. PMID: 32277835; PMCID: PMC7954213.

Fan, L., Chatterjee, S., & Kim, J. (2022). An integrated framework of young adults' subjective well-being: The roles of personality traits, financial responsibility, perceived Financial Capability, and race. *Journal of Family and Economic Issues, 43*(1), 66–85.

Fernańdez-Alcántara, M., García-Caro, M. P., Pérez-Marfil, M. N., Hueso-Montoro, C., Laynez-Rubio, C., & Cruz-Quintana, F. (2016). Feelings of loss and grief in parents of children diagnosed with autism spectrum disorder (ASD). *Research in Developmental Disabilities, 55*, 312–321.

12 The Occupational Wholeness Questionnaire

Farzaneh Yazdani

Box 12.1 Chapter aims

This chapter will cover:

- The process of developing the *Occupational Wholeness Questionnaire*
- The directions of future research

The *Occupational Wholeness Questionnaire (OWQ)* is based on the fundamental concepts of the *MOW* that people *Feel* content as a whole when there is *Harmony* in what they *Do* to *Satisfy* their *Needs* of *Being*, *Belonging* and *Becoming* (see Chapter 2). The idea behind developing the questionnaire is to enhance people's *Self-Awareness* about their state of *Being*, *Belonging*, *Becoming* and overall *OW*. The *OWQ* tool provides opportunity to help people develop *Self-Awareness* as well as to participate in a *MOW*-based intervention. As the *MOW* concepts refer to people's subjective experiences, development of a self-assessment tool is well justified. Through a self-assessment tool of what people do to meet their *Needs* for the *3Bs*, they can be helped to identify the areas of their life that require *Re-thinking* and *Re-planning*. The tool also helps to identify people who may have problems that can be explained and dealt with based on the *MOW*. As *Doings* is at the centre of the *MOW*, the *OWQ* questions were developed to indicate how *Doings* can aid meeting *Being*, *Belonging* and *Becoming*. This chapter presents the steps through which the *OWQ* questionnaire (insert citation for how *OWQ* was created/used) was developed and tested for validity and reliability. The following 15 steps were conducted during the development of the questionnaire:

1 Pool of items extracted from qualitative studies created
2 Items mapped against concepts of the *MOW*
3 Creation of table to indicate what items measure
4 Table sent to eight occupational therapy and occupational science scholars to score the validity
5 Low-scoring items removed
6 Items modified in accordance with feedback
7 Table resent to scholars for re-evaluation
8 High-scoring items redrafted as self-descriptive statements
9 Four-point Likert scale used for questionnaire

DOI: 10.4324/9781003034759-12

Table 12.1 Occupational Wholeness Questionnaire (OWQ) Version II

No. Items	Far below my expectation for satisfaction score 1	Moderately below my expectation for satisfaction score 2	Slightly below my expectation for satisfaction score 3	Meets my expectations for satisfaction score 4	Slightly above my expectation for satisfaction score 5	Far above my expectation for satisfaction score 6
1 What I do helps me be myself						
2 What I do makes me feel good about myself						
3 What I do helps me to see the good things in life						
4 What I do supports my well being						
5 What I do makes me a better person						
6 What I do helps me feel I have choices						
7 What I do helps me to manage my self-care						
8 What I do helps me to discover myself						
9 What I do makes me feel good about life/the world						
10 What I do enables me to have fun						
11 What I do enables me to move ahead in my life						
12 What I do is beneficial for my future growth						
13 What I do makes me change for the better						
14 What I do will bring me closer to my goals						
15 What I do ensures a brighter future for myself						
16 What I do helps me develop as I would like to						
17 What I do makes me feel able to attain my goals						
18 What I do helps me to be part of my community						
19 What I do helps me to find my place in the world						
20 What I do helps me get closer to others						
21 What I do makes me feel I would be missed by my community if I were not there						
22 What I do makes me feel valued by others						
23 What I do helps me to be supported by my community						
24 What I do helps me to feel part of my family						

10   Questionnaire sampled by social media users via Internet
11   Factors analysis used to reduce number of items
12   Second survey implemented through social media
13   Rasch analysis used to shorten questionnaire
14   Resulting questionnaire used to finalize 24 items (see Table 12.1)
15   Six-point Likert scale adopted.

The *OWQ II* questionnaire, at this stage of its development, can be used to show shifts in a helpee's progress towards *Change* before and after a *MOW*-based intervention. Further studies are needed to enhance the quality of the questionnaire and its usability with different populations and for different purposes. On the six-point Likert scale, one registers the lowest level of satisfaction while the highest level is six. Therefore, the lowest possible total score is 24, and the highest total score is 144. The higher the total score of the overall *OW* that is a combination of the scores in three *Being, Belonging* and *Becoming* components indicates the higher level of *OW* that people perceive for themselves. However, there are no cut off points as to what may indicate a low-level *OW* that may be helpful in assessing helpees' need for a *MOW*-based intervention.

The following scenario demonstrates the application of the *OWQ II* with a helpee for identifying their problems (Table 12.2). The first application was used pre-intervention, the second application came at the midpoint of the intervention and the third application was at the end of the intervention. Scenario 12.1 is informed by a real situation in which a pseudonym is used.

Scenario 12.1

Rosa is a 50-year-old artist. She used to be very active and perceived herself as a successful person in her field of work. She was diagnosed with the debilitating illness multiple sclerosis (MS) two years ago following significant/lengthy/in-depth investigation conducted by a team of specialists after she had suddenly experienced extreme weakness in her legs, overall fatigue and visual problems. Rosa's reduced ability to manage her life had a huge impact on her *Well Being*. She started showing signs of depression and lack of interest in many of the things she used to enjoy before. Table 12.2 shows Rosa's *OWQ II* scores when a helper first met her to evaluate her eligibility for a 12-week *MOW*-based intervention. Rosa was asked to score the self-descriptive statements in the light of her *Feeling* and *Thinking* during the previous four weeks. The midway use of the *OWQ II* then was planned for week six into her intervention when she was asked to reflect on her *Feelings* and *Thinkings* during week five. The third and final use of the *OWQ II* was implemented two weeks after ending her *MOW*-based intervention when Rosa was asked to consider the two weeks after her discharge from the intervention (Figure 12.1).

The three total scores reveal significant improvement in almost all *OWQ II* items indicating overall enhancement of Rosa's *OW*. At the beginning, it can be interpreted that Rosa's sense of *Being* was most negatively affected by her health condition, while her perceived sense of *Belonging* was the most positive of the three components. Rosa's sense of *Becoming* and future prospects were perceived negatively. After 12 weeks, Rosa's scores had increased from 33 to 101 points, suggesting that the *MOW*-based intervention had helped her to improve her state of *Being, Belonging, Becoming* and overall *OW*.

Table 12.2 Rosa's OWQ II at Three Points: Prior to, Mid stage and after Two Weeks

No	Items	Pre-intervention score 1 (two weeks before intervention)	Mid-intervention score 2 (week five of intervention)	Post-intervention score 3 (two weeks after intervention)
1	What I do helps me be myself	1	2	4
2	What I do makes me feel good about myself	1	2	3
3	What I do helps me to see the good things in life	1	2	3
4	What I do supports my well being	1	3	5
5	What I do makes me a better person	1	3	5
6	What I do helps me feel I have choices	1	2	4
7	What I do helps me to manage my self-care	1	4	5
8	What I do helps me to discover myself	1	3	5
9	What I do makes me feel good about life/the world	1	2	3
10	What I do enables me to have fun	1	2	3
11	What I do enables me able to move ahead in my life	1	3	4
12	What I do is beneficial for my future growth	3	3	4
13	What I do makes me change for the better	2	2	4
14	What I do will bring me closer to my goals	1	2	4
15	What I do ensures a brighter future for myself	1	2	3
16	What I do helps me develop as I would like to	1	2	3
17	What I do makes me feel able to attain my goals	1	2	3
18	What I do helps me to be part of my community	1	3	5
19	What I do helps me to find my place in the world	1	2	4
20	What I do helps me get closer to others	2	3	5
21	What I do makes me feel I would be missed by my community if I were not there	2	3	4
22	What I do makes me feel valued by others	3	3	5
23	What I do helps me to be supported by my community	2	3	5
24	What I do helps me to feel part of my family	2	5	5
	Total score	33	62	101

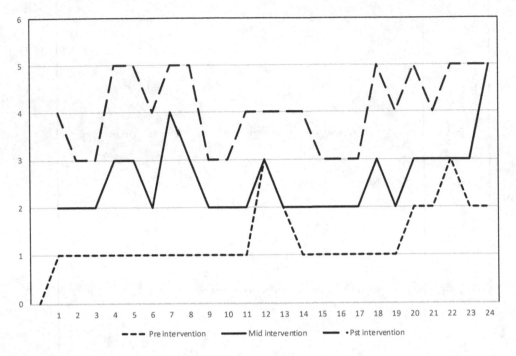

Figure. 12.1 Changes in Rosa's OWQ II Scores

Summary

The development of OWQ II is explained. The example of the application of the OWQ II as a tool for Reflection is provided and the need for further investigation of the tool is presented.

Acknowledgements

The authors would like to thank Dr Ali Asgari, University of Social Welfare and Rehabilitation Sciences, for his advice on developing the *Occupational Wholeness Questionnaire* and Dr Khedar Mate of McGill University for his work on OWQ II.

Further reading

Bonsaksen, T., & Yazdani, F. (2020). The Norwegian occupational wholeness questionnaire (N-OWQ): Scale development and psychometric properties. *Scandinavian Journal of Occupational Therapy, 27*(1), 4–13.

Bonsaksen, T., & Yazdani, F. (2018). Sociodemographic factors associated with the Norwegian occupational wholeness questionnaire scales. *ErgoScience* 13(1), 14–20.

Boone, W. J. (2016). Rasch analysis for instrument development: Why, when, and how? *CBE— Life Sciences Education, 15*(4), rm4.

Boparai, J. K., Singh, S., & Kathuria, P. (2018). How to design and validate a questionnaire: A guide. *Current Clinical Pharmacology, 13*(4), 210–215.

Kang, H. (2013). A guide on the use of factor analysis in the assessment of construct validity. *Journal of Korean Academy of Nursing, 43*(5), 587–594.

Rebeiro Gruhl, K. L., Boucher, M., & Lacarte, S. (2021). Evaluation of an occupation-based, mental-health program: Meeting being, belonging and becoming needs. *Australian Occupational Therapy Journal, 68*(1), 78–89.

13 The MOW scholars and future directions of MOW projects

Farzaneh Yazdani

Box 13.1 Chapter aims

This chapter will cover:

- Introduction to the MOW network (MOWNET)
- The current state of scholarly activities in relation to the *MOW*
- Suggestions for further development of the *MOW*

The MOW network

There are currently several international scholars working together on introducing the *MOW* and applying it in their own field of work (see Figure 13.1). Here are seven of these scholars who shared their work that are presented as scenarios in different chapters. These scholars are part of the *MOW* Network that has an Instagram account. The *MOW* Instagram, which has its own logo (see Figure 13.2), is used as a platform for introducing the *MOW* concepts and is open to the public:

Dr Farzaneh Yazdani (@occupationalwholeness)
https://instagram.com/occupationalwholeness?igshid=MDE2OWE1N2Q=

The current MOW-related projects and scholars

Sarah Kufner (Germany)

I am an occupational therapist. I hold a BSc in Health in Occupational Therapy from the Netherlands and Professional Systemic Coach (DGSF) qualifications from Germany. I am currently studying for an MSc in Health Psychology and Prevention (see Figure 13.3). As a founder of *The Empowerment Project* (www.empowerment-project.de) which started in 2016, I engage in empowering healthcare and education workers in facilitating a more human and just health and educational future. As part of *The Empowerment Project* outreach, we offer themed events and coaching at individual and community levels.

I appreciate discovering different ways of learning and teaching on my journey towards becoming an occupational therapist. In one of my practice fields, I work with children and their families as part of an interprofessional team. These professional collaborations facilitate a multiperspective view of children and their family situations, so I

DOI: 10.4324/9781003034759-13

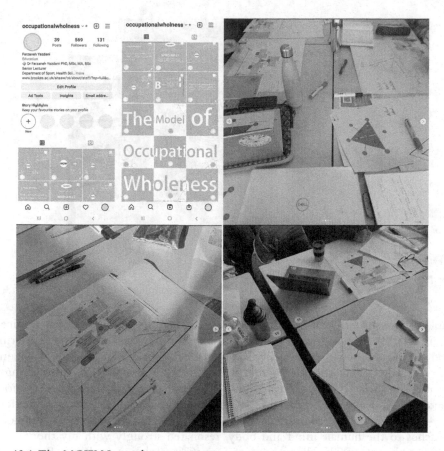

Figure 13.1 The MOW Network

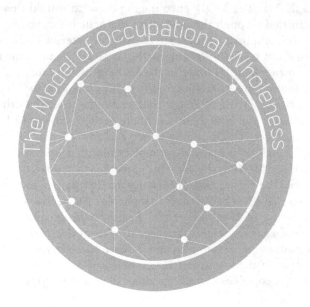

Figure 13.2 The Occupational Wholeness Logo

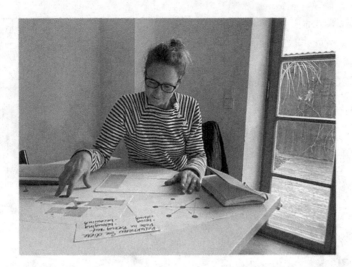

Figure 13.3 Sarah Kufner

am able to provide effective child-centred as well as family-centred therapy service for the families I am working with. Working in a multiprofessional team has furthermore helped me to gain growing experience in understanding and managing team dynamics.

I first learned about the *MOW* in 2017 when reading an article introducing the *Model of Occupational Wholeness* in the online German professional journal *Ergoscience – Advances in Occupational Therapy*. The *MOW's* integrative approach to combination of reality-based therapy and cognitive behavioural therapy, as well as spiritual and holistic approaches to the human mind and body, resonated strongly with my thoughts and mindset at that time. The dimensions of *Doing(s?)* in relation to *Being, Belonging* and *Becoming* illustrated through *Triangles* make the dynamics of an individual's *Doings* come alive. I appreciate the way the *MOW* encourages people to unfold their narratives and how *Change* is facilitated through the interactive dialogue between helper and helpee.

To me, the *MOW's* emphasis on interactive dialogue offers a challenging and joyful process of bringing about *Change*. Working with the *MOW* requires me to be *Self-Aware* and *Reflective* in my own practice. I find that the *MOW* principles are challenging me as an own practice to be focused so as to facilitate clients' *Awareness about* their issues. The *MOW* aids helpees to *Feel* safe by giving them the time and space to identify the links between their *Feelings* and *Thoughts* and how these contribute in their sense of *OW*. *Enabling* clients to *Reflect* on what they *Do/Not Do* and how they *Feel* and *Think* is like watching a bush come into bloom. The *MOW* is really about understanding people and their narratives.

What I like about the *MOW* is the way this model views human beings *Wholeness,* no matter how *Dissatisfied* the person *Feels* or how negatively they perceive themselves at that time in their life. The *MOW* acknowledges that people's perspective of their own life can *Change* as can their sense of *Wholeness*. These *Empowering* principles can bring hope by *Enabling* people to realize that these experiences are part of the natural process of human life. I find the use of drawing *Actual, Ideal* and *Tailored Triangles*, thereby visualizing people's *Doings* in relation to their senses of *Being, Belonging* and *Becoming*, a strong way of raising and enhancing people's *Self-Awareness* about themselves and their life.

I have used the *MOW* on several occasions including in my work with Hannah (see Chapter 6) who is in transition to *Becoming* a young adult. Facing *Change* between stages of her life, Hannah finds it challenging to *Plan* for her future. I thought Hannah may find the *MOW* helpful in *Thinking* and *Reflecting* on her current situation and future plans. Hannah' scenario is presented in Chapter 6: *Planning* the *Change* and a brief account of Sarah's reflection on her work with Hannah is also presented in Chapter 9: *Reflection* as strategy to enhance *Self-Awareness*.

I also used the *MOW* in working with adults in my role as a professional coach. I found the *MOW* useful in assisting my helpees to perceive their current life situation clearly and to *Reflect* on their life. The *MOW Enabled* my helpees to *Become* more *Aware* of the *Disharmonies* in their *Doings* in relation to meeting their *Needs* for *Being, Belonging and Becoming*. It also helped them to identify the factors within their *Context* that were facilitating or blocking their *Choice-Making*. This process of (what?) *Empowered* them to *Become* to be more *Self-Aware* of their *Autonomy* and *Competencies*.

Mehdi Rezaee (Iran)

I am an occupational therapist working in Tehran-Iran. I hold a BSc in Occupational Therapy from the University of Shahid Beheshti, Iran, an MSc and PhD from University of Social Welfare and Rehabilitation Sciences, Iran. I am an academic member of the Department of Occupational Therapy, School of Rehabilitation, Shahid Beheshti University of Medical Sciences, Tehran (see Figure 13.4). I have been working and educating students in the field of mental health since 2001. I became acquainted with the *MOW* through participating in *MOW* workshops and reading related articles, as well as attending the MOW NETWORK discussion sessions with Dr Yazdani.

I have used the *MOW* in working with my clients in mental health settings and been teaching the basic principles and application of the *MOW* to my students since 2021. Based on the feedback I have received from students and clients during this period of over ten years, I believe the model is easily understood and can be used in practice.

Using *Actual* and *Ideal Triangles* was very useful in raising *Self-Awareness* in clients, and developing *Tailored Triangles* was an extremely helpful aid in determining clients' goals. With my clients, we discussed the factors that were affecting the *Change* process. I found the *MOW* a practical model with useful visual aids that help build a collaborative relationship between the helper and helpee. I have used the *MOW* for clients who were cognitively competent and in the future I would like to explore the application of the *MOW* with people who have impaired cognition.

Part of Mehdi's work is presented in Chapter 5 in Ayda's scenario which includes figures of her *Actual* and *Ideal Triangles* (see Scenario 5.3).

Wa'd Abu Zurayk (Jordan)

I am an occupational therapist located in Amman, Jordan. I have been working in the field of paediatrics since 2006. I hold a BSc in Occupational Therapy from the University of Jordan, an MSc in Intellectual (Learning) Disability Studies from the University of Birmingham, UK and a postgraduate certificate in Applied Neuroscience from King's College London, UK (see Figure 13.4). Throughout my professional journey in working at schools, clinics and with non-governmental organizations (NGOs), I realized that I most enjoyed working in early intervention targeting children who

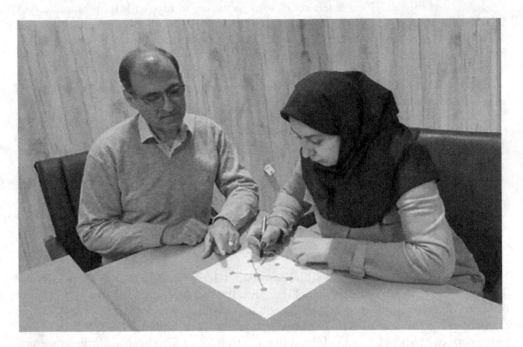

Figure 13.4 Mehdi Rezaee

struggle with challenges caused by mental health and developmental disorders of early childhood.

As part of my work within this field, I facilitate my clients' engagement in their different life roles and occupations. I also provide family support to ensure that the caregivers are *Empowered* with enough skills to promote their child's participation in expected daily living activities in their natural environments. I was introduced to the *MOW* in 2021 as part of my ongoing research work with Dr Yazdani. And while I primarily work in the field of paediatrics, I found a valuable chance to use this model with the parents of my clients. The *MOW* offered an opportunity to help the anxious caregivers who struggled with caring for their children with developmental disabilities, while simultaneously managing other stressful life *Responsibilities* related to their jobs, family lives, etc.

My personal preference as a therapist, when choosing a therapeutic approach, is to select/*Choose* one that allows me to create a narrative of the person's story, including their challenges and highlights. I believe that the best and most *Reflective* story is written in cooperation with the clients themselves. The *MOW* has allowed me to do just that! The significance of the *MOW* is highlighted by the fact that it offers the clinician an opportunity to work in cooperation with their client to explore the origin of their *Dissatisfactions* and anxieties. The *MOW* allows the client to better understand themself and the *Contextual Factors* detracting from their *Satisfaction* in life, through this scientific and focused interaction-based approach that investigates a person's *Choice* of *Doings* to *Satisfy* their psychosocial *Needs* of *Being, Belonging* and *Becoming*. A common issue that tends to arise in my conversations with the families I work with is related to frustrations originating from what they perceive as their limited resources, whether in financial terms or in respect of the support offered by people around them. The *MOW* has helped my clients, called helpees in the language of the *MOW*, and me to put things in context while investigating those "limited" yet often obtainable resources, as well as attach more *Realistic* and *Reflective Meanings* to their different possible *Choices* in *Doings*. With this contextualization, a client is guided through a journey of self-exploration, which commonly leads to a new perception of *Self*, surrounding environment, and a universe of possibilities (Figure 13.5). Wa'd's work with Enas is presented in Chapter 3: Understanding people and their narratives.

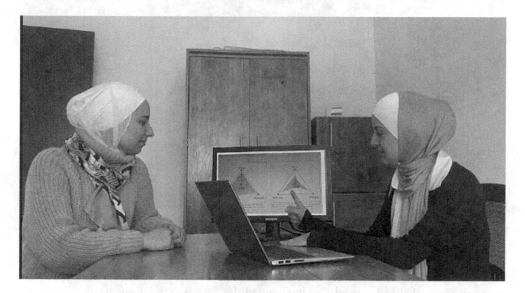

Figure 13.5 Wa'd Abu Zurayk

Nadine Scholz-Schwärzler (Germany)

I have a BSc in Health Occupational Therapy from the Netherlands and an MSc in Occupational Therapy and have been working in (the Netherlands and) Germany with children and their caregivers since 2003 (see Figure 13.6). I have also worked in the other fields of occupational therapy practice including early intervention, curative day care centres and orphanages. I am also interested in and have worked in community-oriented projects. I have been trained in the field of coaching and I am currently a trainer. In 2012, I started working as an occupational therapy lecturer (in Germany) and my role involves teaching, curriculum development and practical tutoring and mentoring prospective occupational therapists. I am grateful to be part of *The Empowerment Project* launched by Sarah Kufner (see above). When I attended the *MOW* workshop, I found the perspective of *Doing/Not Doing* very appealing. I now use the *MOW* in working with my clients and their families. I also use the *MOW* in relation to team work in an organizational *Context*.

As an occupational therapist I accompany people in facing their own assumptions, *Thinking* and *Doings* in their lives. The *MOW Triangles* nicely facilitate this process of self-exploration, by providing *Enabling* tools for *Reflection*. I have used the *MOW* in school settings when working with teenagers and their family members. I have also used

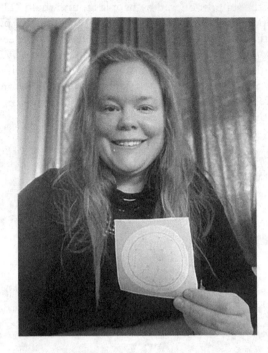

Figure 13.6 Nadine Scholz–Schwärzler

the *MOW* in the educational organization where I work to identify and problem solve our team issues that had caused *Dissatisfaction* with some aspects of our work.

Nadines application of the *MOW* in her workplace and a brief report of her work is presented in Chapter 10: Applying MOW in non-health-related settings.

Melissa Ross Bowen (USA)

I have a BSc in Occupational Therapy, MSc in Psychology, Master of Divinity of Phillips Theological Seminary and Doctor of Occupational Therapy, in progress, Kansas University Medical Center (see Figure 13.7). My occupational therapy practice has included work in a variety of paediatric settings in the USA. I have served as a demonstration teacher at The University of Tennessee and have been the academic fieldwork coordinator for the occupational therapy assistant programme at Baptist Health College Little Rock for 10 years. My current faculty practice includes supervision of an occupational therapy assistant providing out-patient services to adults with developmental disabilities. I am also a part-time minister in The United Methodist Church and serve at a mission church for persons experiencing homelessness, where we provide mentoring and primary medical care. I discovered the occupational justice work of Ann Wilcock in a theory and practice class for my doctoral programme and began reading all I could find. As a minister and an occupational therapist, I felt a great affinity with her work.

After the class ended, I continued to explore the literature that had evolved from Wilcock's original premises and discovered the *MOW* as I was reviewing literature for a lecture on occupational balance. I was thrilled when I got the article because this model

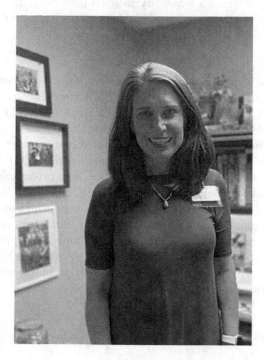

Figure 13.7 Melissa Bowen

includes all the aspects I loved in Wilcock's work and provides a guide for assessment and intervention, which was lacking in other models. I had also been reviewing a variety of models for addressing spirituality in occupational therapy and was disappointed time and again when I discovered a promising model, but it was limited in scope or did not include a framework for assessment and intervention. The *MOW* is both specific enough to provide meaningful direction for the therapeutic process and general enough to be useful across persons and settings.

Dr Yazdani has provided me with her mentorship and additional information as I have developed a group intervention *(Making Meaning)* for persons with progressed multiple sclerosis using the *MOW* to focus on spiritual occupations. This group intervention development has been undertaken as a part of my doctoral capstone research. As both an occupational therapist and clergyperson, I am so excited to use this model which I believe has the capacity to serve us well as a frame to provide occupational therapy targeted toward spiritual occupations. The *MOW* defines *Doing* as a *Need* that helps us meet our other *Needs* for *Being* ourselves, as well as *Becoming,* through the development of *Autonomy* and competence, and *Belonging,* through relationships with other people, places or things. These notions are compatible with my own understanding of spirituality as a journey (or *Becoming*) of *Connection* to the sacred, which can be found both beyond and within the *Self* (*Being*). I believe the spiritual journey may be solitary at times, but it is greatly enriched when shared through deep *Connection* with others and recognition of our *Connection* to the sacred in the world around us (*Belonging*).

At the time of this writing, a feasibility study is underway, and I am looking with great anticipation for how the members of *Making Meaning* respond!

Laya Nobakht (Iran)

I have a BSc and an MSc in clinical psychology from Azad University, Iran. I am a PhD candidate in the field of health psychology, Azad University, Iran (see Figure 13.8). I attended Dr Yazdani's workshop in Tehran about the *MOW* and became interested in the way it looks at public health and promoting *Well Being* from an occupational science perspective. Being familiar with the fundamental theories underpinning the *MOW,* I found its unique way of *Re-thinking* and *Re-planning* life through *Reflection* an engaging collaborative process between the helper and helpee. As a psychologist, I appreciate the emphasis that this model puts on developing narrative collaboratively and raising *Awareness* in helpees about themselves and their life opportunities and limitations. I integrated the philosophy of the model with Rational Emotive Behavioural Therapy that I am trained for. I am in charge of the *MOW* Instagram and social network accounts and enjoy preparing material for them. Collaboration with other *MOW* scholars has given me an opportunity to see the application of the *MOW* from different cultural and language perspectives when preparing the material to post on social media.

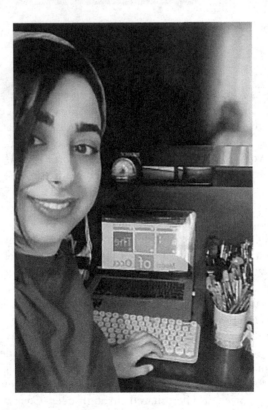

Figure 13.8 Laya Nobakht

Salma Nobakht (Iran)

I have a BA in Graphic Design from University of Science and Culture, Iran, with a special interest in designing art- and music-related posters (see Figure 13.9).

I became interested in health-related posters and educational booklets through Dr Yazdani's work and am grateful that I had an opportunity to design the MOWNET logo and the *MOW* social platform.

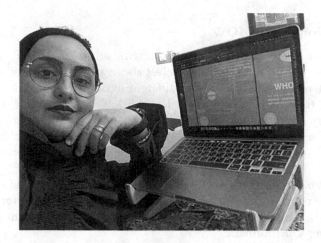

Figure 13.9 Salma Nobakht

Niayesh Fekri (UK)

I am an Iranian–British artist and educator living and working in London. I graduated from the Slade School of Fine Art in 2020. I work in a variety of mediums which include moving-image, writing, bookbinding and performance. The themes in my work often

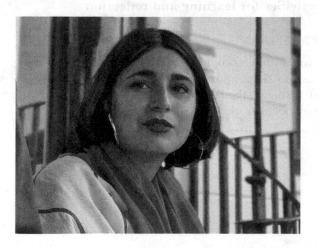

Figure 13.10 Niayesh Fekri

deal with modes of storytelling and conversation to register the fragmentary and ghostly nature of immigrant experiences, familial relationships, fictions and memory. As an educator I work with people of all ages in workshop settings.

In my discussions with Dr Yazdani about the *MOW* book, I was interested to see how case studies and examples can be used to tell stories from a variety of intersectional perspectives. Most importantly, I enjoyed learning about the *MOW* and its capacity for facilitating people's expression of their own *Choices* and their processes of *Meaning-Making* (Figure 13.10).

Future direction of the MOW

The development of the *MOW* which started with studies in 2012 is still at an early stage. The scholars who introduced themselves above are working on the utility of the *MOW* with different populations and in different settings. Readers are invited to join the MOWNET (insert URL, etc., or see details below) to discuss their ideas and feedback their experience of applying the *MOW* to assist with improvement of the model.

Projects to develop further tools and a *MOW*-based app have begun and the scholars hope these tools and app will be able to facilitate the *MOW* application among users in the near future.

The *Occupational Wholeness Questionnaire II* (see Chapter 12) is being reviewed to establish further psychometric qualities to allow the tool to be used for research purposes. The *MOW* scholars have also been working on the development of the General Sense of *Belonging* Questionnaire.

Summary

The *MOW* scholars and their ongoing contribution to the MOW development are presented. The future direction of the *MOW* projects is introduced.

Box 13.2 Activities for learning and reflection

As student or practitioner,

- How do you think you could use the *MOW* in your practice?
- If you wish to share your stories about applying the *MOW* through the MOWNET, contact the Farzaneh Yazdani using the following email address fyazdani@brookes.ac.uk

Index

Note: **Bold** page numbers refer to tables and *italic* page numbers refer to figures.

Abu Zurayk, Wa'd 179–181, *181*

Actual Doings 62–63, 66, 74, 87, 108, 146, 162, 164; *see also* Doing, Not Doing, Doings

Actual Triangles 27, *27*, 52, *53*, *54*, 55, 66, *67–68*, 74, 83, 94, 117, 146, **161**; and COVID-19 pandemic 145–146; creating 62; Disharmony and Incongruence *164*; Incongruence between Ideal Triangles and 57; scoring 66–69; Skewed 52–53

analysis: art of 63–64; of the Incongruence between Actual and Ideal Triangles 78S

Assigning Meaning 6, 22, 54, 125, 160

Assignment of Meaning: negative 21, 22, **72**, **161**; positive 54, **72**, **161**

Attributing Value 4–5, 6, 18, 21, 29, 69, **72**, **161**

Autonomy 5, 9, 16

Awareness 35, 39, 40, 87, 88; about own characteristics 36; helpers' 36; *see also* Self-Awareness

Balance 3, 4, 6, 9, 26; defined 2; and imbalance 2

Becoming 3, 4, 9–11, 19, 21, 64, 78, 118, 136, **161**; Context 23–26; and Dissatisfaction 43; and Doings 108; Harmony/lack of Harmony between Being, Belonging and 57; mothers' poorer sense of 145; sense of 145, 151, 152

Becoming-Belonging 23

Becoming Needs 96, **96**

Being 3, 4, 9–11, 15–16, 19, 21, **161**; Context 23–26; and Dissatisfaction 43; existing needs **95**; Harmony/lack of Harmony between Belonging, Becoming and 57; living needs **95**; Needs for 10, 20, 29, 40, 41, 57, 58, 63, 64, 68, 77, 98, 179; survival needs **95**

Being, Belonging and Becoming (3Bs) *see* 3Bs of Doings

Being-Becoming 22–23, 66, 96

Being-Belonging 14, 22, 66, 96

Belonging 3, 4, 9–11, 16–17, 21, 78, 82, **161**; concepts of 47; Context 23–26; and Dissatisfaction 43; Harmony/lack of Harmony between Being, Becoming and 57; levels 18–19; levels of 95, **95**; Needs 17, 59, 64

Belonging-Becoming 66, 96

Blocking 24, 25, 26, **51**

Borton, T. 125, 131, 133

Bowen, Melissa Ross 182–184, *183*

Capacities 5; and Choices 28; Contextual 9, 80, 131–133, 164; Emotional 9; helpees 40; Individual 3, 65–66, 83, 103, 112, 116, 131, 133

Carlson, D. S. 2

Change(s) 6–7, 8, 29, 34; approaches and methods to helping 103–104; aspects of **98**; and Becoming 19; Change making 93–94; Change process 94–98; conceptualizing 62–69, 160, 162, 165, *165*; intended Change 94; Motivators 82, 116, *117*; natural 9; in people's Context 10; Prediction and Expectation 98–102; Re-Planning principle 93–94, 98; Re-Thinking principle 93–94; starting points of 65; Tailored (Reality) Triangle 92–93

Changeability 6, 97, **161**

Change making: Re-Planning principle 93–94; Re-Thinking principle 93–94

Change process *93*, 94–98; actuating Reflection 94; Doings (Doing/Not Doing) 94; enabling Practice 94; going through 112–121; re-thinking and choice-making 94–98; re-thinking and self-awareness 94–98; Thinking and Feeling 94

Change Profile (activity) 126, *126*

children with disabilities: in Iran 143–144; mothers as carers for 143–144

Choice-Making 4–7, 11, 16, 19, 57, 69, 92, 94–95, 97–98, 95, 120–122, 142, 154, **161**, 179; re-thinking through facilitating 94–98

Choices 5–6, 7, 24, 41, 56; *vs.* Obligation 79; Occupational 29; and personal capacities 28

collage making (activity) 122–123, *123*

college students and MOW 154–156, *155*, *156*

Compassion-Focused Therapy (CFT) 97

compatibility of MOW with other models 147

Congruence 97, 107, **161**

Congruence/Incongruence of the Actual and Ideal Triangles 26–29; *see also* Incongruence

Connectedness 16, 18, 23, 47

Connection 16, 18, 22, 25, 30, 58–59, 81, 95, 183

Context 5, 8, 14, 15, 29, 34–35, 41, 59, 65, 78; Being, Belonging, Becoming and Doings 23–26; of a person's life 5; role of 4–7; and Self-Awareness 9; sense of Being 22

Contextual Capacities 9, 80, 131–133, 164

Contextual Factors 5, 23–24, 65, 103; cards 112, *114*; defined 26; identifying/adjusting/ modifying and replacing 123; negative **161**; positive **161**; Unchangeable 40

Contextual support 101, 133, 145–146, 150–152

Control 6–7, 14–15; locus of 7

COVID-19 pandemic 86, 141–142; MOW in educational settings during 150–152; public interpretation of responses to 142–143

Cutchin, M. P. 20

Del Fabro Smith, L. 15

Demanding 24, 25, **51**

Demands 19, 24, 28, 34, 55, 59, 93; of modern life 4; multiple 2

Demotivation 6, 20–22, 78, 148

Devil-Angel board game (activity) 116, *116*

Discrepancy 160, 164, *164*; *see also* Gap

Disharmony **161**; identifying 160, 164, *164*

Dissatisfaction 6, 17, 34, 42, 52, 66, 68, 79, 86, 88, 102, 145, 148, 152, 156, 160, 180, 182; group activities the areas of 88; identifying indicators of 42–43; MOW used for exploring 86–87; types of 43

Doing, Not Doing, Doings 3–4, 6–7, 9–11, 14, 19–21, 23, 34, 59, 66, 74, 94, **161**; and 3Bs 88; Context 23–26; defined 20; individual's 80; Intentional 19–20; Meaning Assigned to 20–21; Meaning of 24; Motivation for 56–57; MOW-based analysis of Sally's **99**; Planned 19; Voluntary 20

Doings-Becoming 96

Doings-Being 94–95

Doings-Belonging 95

Doings Cards *114*

drawing the balloon person (activity) 111–112, *111*

Emotion(s) 8, 17, 94, 118, 121

Emotional Capacities 9

Emotional Value 18, 20

empathy 40–41, 97

Empowering 40, 41, 50, 81, 92, 103

The Empowerment Project 176, 181

Enablers 41

Enabling strategies 40

Encouraging 24, 25, 40, **51**, 103

encouraging strategies 40–42, 168

Ergoscience – Advances in Occupational Therapy 178

Expecting 24, 25, **51**, 59

experience of people 36–38

Explore-Predict (E-P) card playing (activity) 112–115, *113–115*

Facilitating 24, 25, 39, **51**, 69

Feeling Change diagram 118, 120, *120*

Feelings 94; acknowledging/validating and monitoring 118–119; cards *112*; Empowered 104

Fekri, Niayesh *185*, 185–186

final summative Reflection 163, 166

Gap 2, 4, 27, 55, 57, 160, 164, *164*; *see also* Incongruence

Gibbs model 131, 132

Happiness 2, 5, 95; defined 3; and life satisfaction 3; *vs.* satisfaction 3

Harmony 3–4, 8, 9, 27, 29, 52, 55, 77–78, **161**, 170; between Being and Becoming 57–59; lack with Belonging 57–59

Harmony/lack of Harmony: between Being, Belonging and Becoming 57; between Being and Becoming 57–59

Health: and MOW 7–8; and Well Being 7–8

Health Belief (HB) model 147–148

helpees: Capacities 40; communication, responding effectively to 40; evaluating an individual Readiness for MOW-based intervention 71–74; examples of 42; and helpers interaction 43–47; MOW concepts and suggested questions to ask **51**; narratives 38–39; Needs 40; Readiness for Change 71–90; Reflection 132; strategies for progress of interaction between helper and 40; verbal and non-verbal language 40

Helper-Helpee collaborative Reflection 132, 134–136; action plan 135; analysis 135; description 134; evaluation 134; feelings and thoughts 134; Now What? 136; So What? 136; What? 136

helper-helpee relationship 36, 39, 41–42

helpers: educational strategies 41–42; encouraging strategies 41; extra skills in developing public-level project 90; and helpee interaction 43–47; identifying resources 85; in-depth interaction with helpee 39; Reflection 132–134, 137; strategies for progress of interaction between helpees and 40; strategies to empathize 41

human development process 1

Human Needs: and MOW 4; *see also* Needs

Hypothetical Actual and Ideal Triangles 27, *27*

Ideal Doings 74

Ideal Triangles 27, *27*, 52, *53*, *54*, 55, 66, *67–68*, 74, 83, 146, **161**; creating 62, 77–78; group activities to facilitate understanding 88; Incongruence between Actual Triangles and 57; scoring 66–69

Imaginary Activity 121, *121*

Imbalance 3–5, 6, 9; and balance 2; defined 2

Incongruence 83, 107, **161**; between Actual and Ideal Triangles, analysis of 78; degree of 54–55; group activities the areas of 88; large degree of 55; and Meaning-Making 54–55; Meaning-Making impact on 56; small degree of 55; *see also* Gap

Individual Capacities 3, 65–66, 83, 103, 112, 116, 131, 133

Individual Intervention Decision-Making Chart 73, *73*

Inhibiting 24

intended change 94

Intention 14–15, 20

Intentional Purpose 20

Intentional Relationship Model 36

interpersonal characteristics 36

interpretation, art of 63–64

Jensen, S. Q. 18

knowledge of people 36–38

Kofodimos, J. R. 2

Kufner, Sarah 139, 176–179, *178*, 181

Life Balance 2–3; from MOW perspective 3–4

life development 31–32

Life Dissatisfaction 7

Life Satisfaction 5, 8, 11; and balancing doings 4; and happiness 3; and imbalancing doings 4

Like/Dislike Change activity 120, *121*

Meaning 5; assigning 6, 20–21; assigning negative 21

Meaning Assignment 5, 20–21

Meaningfulness 20

Meaning-Making 4–7, 11, 16, 21–22, 28, 54–55, 69, 92, 94; impact on Incongruence 56; negative **161**; positive **161**

Model of Occupational Wholeness (MOW) 2, 14–31, 50, 178; -based analysis of Sally's Doings **99**; -based problem identification 87–88; Change, conceptualizing 160, 162, 165, *165*; and college students 154–156, *155*, *156*; components 10–11, *11*; concepts and suggested questions to ask helpees **51**; concepts in lay language **72**, **161**; COVID-19 pandemic 142–143; Disharmony, Discrepancy/Gap 160, 164, *164*; in educational settings during pandemic 150–152; employing, in workplace 152–154, *153*; final summative Reflection 163, 166; goal of 9–10; and health 7–8; Health Belief (HB) model 147–148; interaction-centred intervention in 39; intervention 40, 42, 92; in non-health-related settings 141–157; people and narratives 160, 164; person's Readiness for Change 162, 165; perspective, life balance from 3–4; principles of 28–29, 146–147; projects 176–186; in public level 84–89; public narratives 145–146; and quality of life 8; rule of 'SEVEN' 160–163; scholars 176–186; SoBC model 149–150; strategies 162–163, 166; and Well Being 7–8, 146; wholeness clock 149, *149*

"Model of Reflection" 125, 131, 133, 135–136

mothers: as carers for children with disabilities 143–144; of children with disabilities Well Being 146

Motiva(tion, tional, or motive) 6–7, 10, 20–21, 34, 41, 47, 54, 56–57, 82, 116, *117*

MOW-based intervention 28, 34, 37, 40, 42, 62, 66; individual helpee's Readiness for 71–79, 81

MOW Network (MOWNET) 176, *177*

narratives: collage making (activity) 122–123; developing 121; people and their 160, 164; public 145–146

Needs 14, 26, 39; for Being 10, 20, 28, 29, 40, 41, 57, 58, 63, 64, 68, 77, 98, 179; Belonging 17, 59, 64; helpees 40, 41; psychological 9; survival 2; of target group 85; types of 3; *see also* Wants
Negative Thoughts 145
Nobakht, Laya 184, *184*
Nobakht, Salma 185, *185*
non-health-related settings: MOW in 141–157
Not Belonging 17–18

objectively identified problems: *vs.* perceived experience 57; *vs.* subjective experience 57
Obligations 88, 97, **161**; *vs.* Choices 79
Occupational Balance 2–3
occupational therapists 11, 143, 145
Occupational Wholeness (OW) 2, 15, 50, **161**; components of the sense of 15–21, 23, 30–31; Triangles of 26–28, *27*
Occupational Wholeness Questionnaire (OWQ) 170–174, **171**, **173**, *174*; Version II **171**, 172, 186
Occupational Wholeness Questionnaire (OWQ) II **171**, 172, 186; prior to, mid stage and after two weeks **173**; scores *174*
Opportunity 24–26, 30, 34, 40, 59
Opposing 24–25, **25**
'othering' 18

perceived experience 57
picture/film watching (activity) 119
Planned Change: acting on 118; as strategy for Change 118
Planning 20, 23; strategies 162, 166
Practising, as strategy for Change 124
Predicting 6, 10, 22, 23
Prediction/Expectation 98–102; card board *99*
Predictor values 10
public interpretation of responses to pandemic 142–143
public narratives 145–146
Purpose 20–21, 22

quality of life, and MOW 8

Readiness 92, 139, 162
Readiness for Change: creating Ideal Triangles 62, 77–78; creating the Actual Triangle 74–77; helpees 71–90; identifying person's 162, 165; Incongruence between Actual and Ideal Triangles 78; individual's *Doings* 80; individual's views 79–80

real encounter activity 121
Reality Triangle **161**
Reciprocity of Feeling 18
Reflection/Reflecting 102, 107; 3W diagram (activity) 125, *125*, 126; activities for 104; Change Profile (activity) 126, *126*; final summative 163, 166; Helpee's 132; Helper-Helpee collaborative 132, 134–136; Helper's 132–134; in relation to Thinking-Feeling-Doings 125; strategies to help with 137–138; as strategy for Change 125–128; as strategy to enhance Self-Awareness 130–140; types of 138–140; vignette cards (activity) 127, *127–128*; 'What?, So What? Now What?' approach 125, *125*
Relatedness 16, 18
Re-Planning 92, 93–94, 98
Responsibilities 7, 79; for Change process 92
Restricting 24, 25, **51**
Re-Thinking 92; and choice-making 94–98; Doings-Becoming 96; Doings-Being 94–95; Doings-Belonging 95; principle 93–94; and self-awareness 94–98; Triangle of Occupational Wholeness 96–98
reversing seats activity 107–111, *108–110*
Rezaee, Mehdi 179, *180*
Rotter, J. B. 7
rule of 'SEVEN' 160–163

Satisfaction 3, 14, 17, 34, 57; Feeling of 16; *vs.* happiness 3
Satisfaction with Life (SWL) 3, 4, 6, 8, 57, 150
Scholz-Schwärzler, Nadine 181–182, *182*
Self-Awareness 29, 39, 50, 63, 78, 103; and contextual circumstances 9; development of 35; helpee's level of 74; Imaginary Activity 121, *122*; Like/Dislike Change activity 120, *121*; and personal circumstances 9; raising 120; real encounter activity 121; reflection as strategy to enhance 130–140; re-thinking through enhancing 94–98; significance of 8–9; as strategy for Change 120
self-exploration: drawing the balloon person (activity) 111–112, *111*; reversing seats activity 107–111, *108–110*; strategies for 106–107; as strategy for Change 106–112
Self-Fulfilment 6, 8, 11, 34, 57
Skewed Actual Triangles 52–53, 59–60
Skewed Triangle **161**
Social Belonging Needs 17
space 24
Speech and Language Pathologists 143

Stage of Behaviour Change (SoBC)
model 149–150, 167; action stage 150;
contemplation stage 150; maintenance stage
150; pre-contemplation stage 149–150;
preparation stage 150; relapse stage 150
strategies: to help with Reflection 137–138;
implementing 162–163, 166; planning
162, 166
strategies for Change: acknowledging/
validating and monitoring Feelings 118–119;
acting on Planned Change 118; change
process 112–121; developing narrative
121; identifying/adjusting/modifying
and replacing Contextual Factors 123;
implementing 106–128; Practising 124;
raising Self-Awareness 120; Reflection
125–128; Self-Exploration 106–112
subjective experience 57
Subjective Well Being (SWB) 4, 8, 11
Suikkanen, J. 3
Supporting 24, 25, **51**
Survival Needs 2

Tailored (Reality) Triangle 83–84, 92–93, 103,
107, 122, *123*, 126, 130, 133, 136, 145–151,
161, 164, 178–179; characteristics of 93;
creating 92–93
Taylor, R. R. 40
Thinking 92; cards *113*; and Change process
114; helpee's capacities for 103; ineffective
95, 96; logical 94; wishful 148, 149
3Bs of Doings 11, 14, 19, 30, 50, 59, 62–63,
88, 93–94, 108, 110, 114, 118, 125, 136,
141–142, 149, 160, 166, 170, 172,
178–180

3W diagram (activity) 125, *125*, 126
Togetherness 16, 18
Triangle of Human Occupational Wholeness
26–28, *27*
Triangle of Occupational Wholeness 96–98
Triangles 10–11, *11*; Actual (*see* Actual
Triangles); Ideal (*see* Ideal Triangles); of
Occupational Wholeness 26–28, *27*

Unchangeable Contextual Factors 40
Unhappiness 6, 7, 52; MOW used for exploring
86–87; *see also* Dissatisfaction
Unrealistic Expectations 7, 93

Value(s) 5, 23, 65; community 25; negative 20;
positive 20
vignette cards (activity) 127, *127–128*
Voluntary 20

Wants 2–3, 17, 39, 65; *see also* Needs
Well Being 4–5, 59, 85; and MOW 7–8;
Subjective 8
Well Being Project 100; of mothers of children
with disabilities 146; principles of 146–147
'*What?, So What? Now What?*' approach 125,
125
What/So-What card sort activity 116–118
Whole Life Satisfaction Theory of Happiness 3
Wholeness 11, 14
wholeness clock 149, *149*
Wilcock, Ann 15, 182–183
workplace, employing MOW in 152–154, *153*
World Health Organization 142

Zimbardo, P. 7

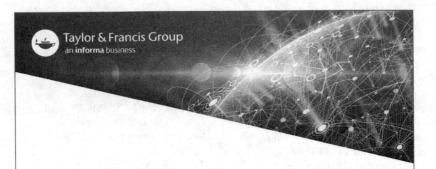